Never Argue *with a*
MATRON

Never Argue *with a*

MATRON

Adventures in Twentieth-Century Nursing

MARY SANDILANDS

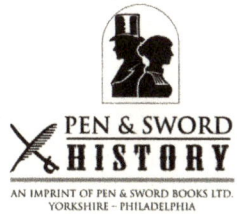

PEN & SWORD
HISTORY

AN IMPRINT OF PEN & SWORD BOOKS LTD.
YORKSHIRE – PHILADELPHIA

First published in Great Britain in 2025 by
PEN AND SWORD HISTORY
An imprint of
Pen & Sword Books Ltd
Yorkshire – Philadelphia

ISBN 978 1 03611 463 3

Typeset in Times New Roman 11.5/14.5 by
SJmagic DESIGN SERVICES, India.
Printed and bound in the UK by CPI Group (UK) Ltd.

Pen & Sword Books Limited incorporates the imprints of Atlas, Archaeology,
Aviation, Discovery, Family History, Fiction, History, Maritime, Military,
After the Battle, Military Classics, Politics, Select, Transport, True Crime,
Air World, Frontline Publishing, Leo Cooper, Remember When,
Seaforth Publishing, The Praetorian Press, Wharncliffe Local History,
Wharncliffe Transport, Wharncliffe True Crime and White Owl.

For a complete list of Pen & Sword titles please contact
PEN & SWORD BOOKS LIMITED
George House, Units 12 & 13, Beevor Street, Off Pontefract Road,
Barnsley, South Yorkshire, S71 1HN, England
E-mail: enquiries@pen-and-sword.co.uk
Website: www.pen-and-sword.co.uk

or

PEN AND SWORD BOOKS
1950 Lawrence Rd, Havertown, PA 19083, USA
E-mail: uspen-and-sword@casematepublishers.com
Website: www.penandswordbooks.com

Contents

Acknowledgements

WITHOUT THE HELP of family and friends this book would never have reached Pen and Sword.

My sister, Jenny Colls, suggested I should publish the two notebooks full of tales of my nursing career, so what began as a memoir for friends and family is now available for a wider readership.

Thank you, Jenny and the many friends who have come to my aid:

Lisa Robinson, who typed the first half.
Claire and Frank Rizos for computer help.
Jean Ainsley and Guy Knight, helpful neighbours.
Joan Kemp, for enormous practical and moral support.
Mary Withall, local friend and author, for advice.
Margaret Webster and Hugo Londoño of Oban Photographic Shop, for transforming photographs.
Paul Brady of Matrix, Oban, for last minute crucial repair of laptop.
Sarah-Beth Watkins, of Pen and Sword, for encouragement and advice.
Karyn Burnham, copyeditor of Pen and Sword, for most helpful suggestions and script changes.

Not many names appear in this narrative, for three reasons:

First is my abysmal memory for names.
Second, they would not mean anything to my family and local friends for whom these tales were originally written.
Third, now that all is to be published, there will less cause for concern about libel laws!

Chapter 1

The Wingfield-Morris Orthopaedic Hospital Headington, Oxford

1953–1955

How unwise to argue with a matron before meeting her.
How unwise at any time… .

APPLYING FOR AN interview when 16 years old, for Orthopaedic training, which could begin at 17, Matron refused, saying that I was too young and might change my mind. Having wanted to be a nurse since the age of 3, this reply was infuriating. My mother, who was an excellent letter writer, wrote again. I was interviewed and accepted, though it was not the last time we clashed.

From the age of 3 I knew I wanted to be a nurse or a teacher. One week at primary school was all it took to remove teacher from my options. After that my only concern for several years was whether wartime clothing restraints and coupons would mean the loss of cloaks, and frilly cuffs from nurses' uniforms.

At 7 years old I had a little table in my grandparents' dining room from which I sold things to friends and family, making £1 for Paulton Hospital. (Somerset). This pleased the grown-ups so much that the following year I had a table at the hospital fete which made more money, though the exact sum is forgotten. From then on it was a case of any excuse to get inside hospitals. I loved them.

1

Several girls at school belonged to St John's Ambulance Brigade cadets, but I never had the slightest inclination to join them. Partly because their classes sounded dull, chiefly because they seemed to have little relevance to hospitals.

When I was 16, on holiday in Somerset with my grandparents but not my parents, a posse of aunts, and especially uncles, began to taunt me about being a nurse, citing all the dreadful things that would happen. I countered each suggestion until, losing my temper, I told them they could say what they liked but I *was* going to be a nurse, and marched out slamming the door. A roar of laughter followed me. It has always been easy to wind me up. Actually the entire family was delighted by my intention and supported me every inch of the way. It was impossible to imagine how girls who had opposition from their parents coped, but some certainly did.

Support did not stop someone once remarking that I might put a patient on a bedpan one day and forget to take them off. Maybe that remark deserved more than laughter. Only once, many years later, did I forget a patient on a bedpan, but nurses with poor memories are a perfect nuisance, and mine was always a bit unreliable.

Also when 16, I knew I did not want to stay at school until I was 18. One year in the sixth form would be quite enough. However, most training schools did not accept girls until they were 18, and St Thomas's, my choice, 19 years. Our family doctor had the solution. Two years at the Wingfield Morris Orthopaedic Hospital. Girls could go there at 17 and nearly all of them went on to do their general training in London – in those days the big London teaching hospitals were regarded as the crème de la crème – furthermore, it was a 'gentle let-down' into nursing as there was no casualty department admitting injured people, and deaths were rare.

After the initial upset about being given an interview, and then having been accepted, I arrived at Pollock House, Jack Straw's Lane, Headington, a suburb of Oxford, in the early afternoon of 14 August 1953, taken by my father; I was 17 years and 48 days old. Having said farewell to my parents and little sister, expecting to be committed to life in the Preliminary Training School for the next five weeks at least, I was back home an hour and a half later. Luckily home was only three miles away.

Our first task had been to sew our Cash's name tapes into our new uniforms. Mine were not in my case – I thought my mother had packed them, she thought I had. Living at the far end of Headington, with Pollock House at the other extreme, it was lucky for me that our notoriously dreadful bus service was cooperative that afternoon, and it was not too long before I joined all the others in the sitting room, stitching and getting acquainted. They were thrilled that my home was in Oxford, and saw me, and Rosemary who also lived locally, as their entrée to university life and undergraduates. Twelve months later I was the only one in our set of twenty-two girls who had never been out with an undergraduate. Before going into the woes of my training let me say that with hindsight my mental age was not a day over 15, and with a naivety which lasted many years after qualifying. Most firmly I believe that no one should start nurse training before 18 years old.

In my last year at school I had done a Pre-Nursing Course, proving yet again useless at Maths but otherwise of middle ability. English and History were always my best subjects – not much good for nursing, but I started well in PTS with an essay on Ethics. It was set during our first week and I came top of the class. After that it was downhill all the way. Well, nearly. Unfortunately, my practical efforts were slow and clumsy, though on my second day of ward experience my polishing of the wooden locker tops in 'the Vatican' – the babies' room in Nani Ward – earned me a pat on the back.

My sketchy diary during this six weeks of PTS details far more social life than study, and though not relevant to this tale of training, reminds me of an amusing (to me) outcome. At this stage youth club was still important, because all our evenings were free so it was possible to go. My roommate often came with me, and also came home with me once or twice. She took me to her home for the long weekend off we were given at the end of PTS, and it was most enjoyable, though her hotelier parents were constantly busy. We happily kept ourselves occupied while assiduously avoiding any hotel guests, as strictly instructed. Back at the hospital after this pleasant weekend, Janey. told me that she had been ordered to have no more to do with me. As a member of a youth club I was not suitable to be a friend.

The club in question was a church Youth Fellowship, run by a gifted family man who was an Oxford graduate and international businessman.

The vast majority of members were day pupils at the local public and grammar schools, and it was considered the best youth club in the city – out of some forty-five. For example, one of the many visits arranged for us had been to the Oxford Union to listen to a debate. For me, the Youth Fellowship gave me many friends, hours of fun, and education.

Hospital duty hours soon meant less attendance and gradually I lost touch with, but never gratitude for, the many and varied activities of almost three years. From tennis to play readings and performances, to quizzes and helping take Evensong at local country churches, we would have been dumbfounded to be considered part of the 'boring' 1950s', let alone 'unsuitable'. The curate who helped with many of our activities ended his career as Archbishop of York. Unsuitable to know??

Years later, a faint thought crossed my mind. The hospital was in the parish of the church I attended, and our vicar was the hospital chaplain. Occasionally, special services for the patients would be held in the hospital gym, and Youth Fellowship members would push beds from the wards down the covered way to the gym. I loved doing that, but it meant that my face was at least vaguely known to staff, my local connection obvious – could there have been some prejudice? Probably not, just my fanciful imagining, yet a tiny glimmer of the idea persists – another reason for my strongly held conviction that everyone should go away from their home area for training or university.

Of course I did for my general training, but that is another story.

Apart from PTS introductory hours, my first ward was Randle; a typical, unheated, one-wall-of-folding-glass-doors easily opened to the elements, classic Wingfield square-shaped ward.

The hospital was built to treat all diseases and deformities of bones. Ortho-paedic = straight-children. When it was founded in the 1920s by far the biggest cause of problems was tuberculosis. Fresh air was an integral part of treatment, and in Randle our day started at 7.30 am with making all the beds. The doors were opened wide during this and nurses were not allowed to wear cardigans. It was a cold autumn.

No coats by the way, though cloaks were issued to night staff. Our caps were made up, quite easily, from an oblong starched piece of flat linen, folded to fit round our heads and with a long straight tail at the back

Short hair, or a bun, off the face. Absolutely no jewellery, not even a wrist watch – that was kept inside a pocket. Fob watches (dreadful things) did not exist. Wedding rings were not even a consideration since nurses had to leave the profession on marriage. It was an absolute that no girl could be committed to the demands of nursing as well as those of marriage and family life. Not only did we wear black shoes and stockings, the shoes had to be bought at a certain shoe shop in Kensington, London. We washed our own stockings but the rest of the uniform went to the hospital laundry. Jewellery and wool, especially cardigans, were considered dangerous, as harbingers of infection and, in the case of jewellery, also as potentially dangerous to the wearer. The simplest stud earring has been known to result in an ear lobe being torn off, and I once worked with a staff nurse who lost a finger when her ring was touched by a diathermy knife (heated by an electric current running through it) in the operating theatre. There must have been some very careless misuse of it by someone!

Randle was a children's ward for boys aged 4 to 7 years, though we did have three girls too. Their beds were in four rows of six, the two central rows back to back. TB, bones and Perthes Disease – a disease of the hip joint, mainly in boys aged 5 to 10 years (mainly pain-free, but untreated would cause a permanent deformity and consequent limp). These were the main problems, keeping the children in hospital for many months. Several were flat on their backs on iron frames, lying on padded leather. Boys with Perthes had weighted leg extensions on one or both legs confining them to bed. Sister had been there for thirty years and was also in charge of the next door ward for girls 8 to 16 years old.

She was terrifying. Teenage reading of hospital stories perhaps influenced my expectations, but she had the same effect on everybody, including qualified staff nurses. Her much younger charge nurse – i.e. both general and orthopaedically qualified – was inclined to be in the same mould. Sister was a woman with a severe squint, rigid physique and not a glimmer of kindness or humour. I did not even have any respect for her. The children had school lessons every day during which their teacher was in charge. After she finished we were instantly expected to keep them quiet. There were not even five minutes in twenty-four hours when they were officially allowed to let off steam, though in most ways they were fit and normal. It seemed barbaric to me but we were always in trouble for not keeping them quiet. Far less important, but still memorably stupid, was the daily polishing of a wooden draining board. This outlandish practice followed the washing of miles of crepe bandages every afternoon, but this was obviously not hospital policy since it did not happen anywhere else.

The bandages accrued during the morning bath times. In a warm room between the two wards each child had a bath once a week. The routine included renewing bandages on the frames and extensions. Not too bad on the straight bits, but on the frames never did I manage it correctly round and through the 'eyes'. It was such a nightmare I used to work out at the beginning of each week how many mornings off I would have and whether there was any possibility of escaping bathing anyone on a frame. Another girl from my set and I were Sister's last new nurses before she retired so at least no on else would ever have to suffer her.

My colleague was bold and buxom, full of self-confidence and although she disliked the ward she had no difficulty with the work. Timid and slow, I remember taking forty minutes to prepare one orange for tea-time! I have no idea how I survived. Not surprisingly, after nine weeks I was given a bad ward report, seen by Matron and sent to work on Burrows, a men's ward.

Sister there had a sister. Both of them had also been in the hospital for thirty years and had formidable reputations, Burrows' Sister less so than the other, who was in charge of the teenage boys' ward. Luckily I got on with her reasonably well. It is true to say that I was automatically afraid of all ward sisters at the Wingfield with perhaps one exception, but none of them were as dreadful as the first.

Burrows was a happy ward. The men were not going to be intimidated.

Christmas was a surprise. Few patients were discharged and all the nurses were on duty all day. However, a side room was organised for staff, with chairs, drinks and nibbles, and we were sent off in twos and threes to visit the other wards all of which, like ours, had Christmas trees and decorations. As usual lunch was served from a hot trolley, each plate individually organised by Sister according to her perception of each patients' appetite or dietary need.

Not as usual, the menu was a traditional one of turkey with all the trimmings, and the turkey was carved by one of the senior surgeons. Father Christmas visited and gave each patient a present and the general atmosphere all day was wonderful.

It was the first of more than a decade of brilliant hospital Christmases for me. It was also the first of many years in which I joined innumerable nurses singing carols round the wards on Christmas Eve, quite late in the evening after the patients were settled and the ward lights dim. A few people carried lanterns, those with cloaks wore them inside out because the linings were red, and outside the babies' ward we always sang 'Away in a Manger'.

In those days it was unheard of for nurses to 'live out', but due to room problems, Matron, with great reluctance, had asked me to live at home for a fortnight over the Christmas period. Home was only a six-minute cycle ride away so it was not a problem and certainly did not prevent me going to the nurses' Christmas dinner. Presided over by Matron, but greatly relaxed due to the levity and antics of a few junior doctors who were present.

Even in those days one heard complaints about 'off-duty', especially mornings off – i.e. 10.30 am to 1 pm, though I never understood why. I always enjoyed variety and being away from the Nurses' Home made no difference. Except that I did not get breakfast in bed on days off! The only Nurses' Home in my experience where that happened.

The 'off-duty' book was the most important in any ward. Requests were virtually unheard of. Later, in other hospitals, requests could at least be written in the book, though never with any guarantee of success. We had one day off weekly and a half-day once a month, always before a day off. Day duty began at 7.30 am and ended at 8 pm. The disliked mornings off actually began at 10.00 am as one went to second coffee. In those supposedly uncivilised days we all had half-hour coffee breaks away from the wards and we also had an hour for lunch. Afternoons off – 2 pm to 5 pm – actually began at 1 pm as one went to second lunch, and evenings began at 5 pm. Tea break for those who had been off in the morning was half an hour. All coffee and meals had two sittings, in order to fit in with ward staffing and the off-duty rotas.

It should not need saying that no ward would ever be left without any staff, hence all the care to ensure proper staffing levels at all times. (An infinitely more difficult task nowadays (2024)).

Apart from the half-day, an evening off always preceded a day off. Night duty, three months at a time, once during our first year, and ditto the second year, twelve nights on then three off. It was rumoured that fifteen on, followed by nine, could happen, though rarely. As a senior nurse I did nine so then expected fifteen on the next rota. Imagine my surprise at only nine for the second time. In fact it was the end of twelve nights for ever, but in those days we were never told anything concerning administration.

In PTS we were taught nothing of the male genitourinary system, it was simply ignored and the male anatomy was not alluded to in the practical classroom. Came the day on Burrows when Sister told me to go and blanket bath Mr A. He was a pleasant middle-aged man with one leg in a long plaster. He was well enough to wash himself apart from his back and reaching the foot of his plastered leg. Anyway I solemnly did his back, front, each arm, free leg and he was equally serious. I hope I let him wash his own face. Certainly when all else was done I panicked, threw the flannel to him and said 'And you can do the rest yourself'. By coincidence – with which my life abounds – between including this bath tale in a rough list and actually writing it, I read Ian McEwan's *Atonement*. Imagine my surprise on reading about nurse training during the war and specifically about the procedure for blanket bathing male patients. And the phrase was 'finish off for himself'. Ian McEwan was only born in 1948 – did a member of his family brief him? No wonder he is an acclaimed author, his descriptions are brilliant as well as accurate.

While on Burrows my unreliable memory played up at least twice. On two occasions I answered the phone, took a message from a houseman and then forgot to pass it on to staff nurses. Surprisingly, mild irritation rather than real annoyance seemed to be the reactions when my misdemeanours came to light.

After a few relatively happy weeks on Burrows I was sent to Gibson, a women's ward. Diary entry for the first day reads: 'Ghastly on Gibson: Burrows seems like heaven in comparison.' But four days later: 'Much better day on ward. Quite bearable in fact.' I was there for three weeks and quite enjoyed it but have one abiding memory: mid-morning bedpans.

Explanation of another nightmare. Bedpan rounds were done after breakfast, lunch, before evening visiting hour and before being settled for the night. Beds were screened using heavy, wooden-framed screens lifted around by hand, they had no wheels – curtains around each bed were a long way in the future. Bedpans were carried by hand to and fro from the sluice always covered by a cloth. Worse were the large, oblong, fairly shallow enamel trays, needed for women lying flat on their backs immobilised in body-fitting plaster beds. These beds were fixed to a frame which in turn sat on a bed and the trays were slipped in underneath. Before use, the cut away plaster behind the patient's bottom had to be stuffed with tow to prevent back-flow. Tow, described in the dictionary as 'prepared fibres of flax, hemp or jute, esp. separated shorter fibres', was brown, fibrous, water-resistant stuff disliked by all. The tangled mess was harsh, sometimes even scratchy, but a far softer, more efficient brown cotton wool was considered too expensive for all but the most seriously ill, usually post-operative, patients. The bedpan ritual, not surprisingly, was time consuming.

Conformity was expected of patients as well as staff and bedpan requests outside the appointed times were not approved of, and junior nurses not encouraged to acquiesce. However, the patients had mid-morning coffee and the 'damp-dusting' routine began soon afterwards. Ward maids did the main cleaning, floors etc., but nurses damp-dusted equipment and locker tops – literally using damp dusters to prevent dust flying around.

I soon came to dread dusting in Room Two. The plea 'May I have a bedpan?' would lead to four or five requests, all from women with complicated beds or splints. The patients, of course, knew which nurses were likely to be prevailed upon. Though not actually chastised, I was frowned on by senior staff for agreeing, but despite taking up to half an hour it still seemed to me more important than dusting. Fifty years on it still does. (Note to MSA sufferers: the dusting still got done, albeit in a hurry).

After a holiday my next ward was Nani, small and warm, for babies and children up to 4 years old. I like children and usually get on well with them, but Sister was a different kettle of fish. With a halo of snow-white hair she was another who had worked in the hospital for thirty years. She knew me by sight from church and I knew her. Austere of expression whether in church or ward, she was the only sister I ever encountered who gave an impression of disliking me as a person. When not ignoring me, nothing I did was right. She was annoyed when once I succeeded with doing a difficult treatment on a 4 year old boy, with whom a staff nurse had battled in vain. She told me the only thing I was any good at was polishing the locker tops. Once she told me she could never find me

9

and to this day I wish I had had the courage to ask her where she thought I was, and tell her she had only to look; it was a small ward, and although it had four interconnecting rooms, I was not given to hiding in the linen cupboard. Talking of small rooms, fast forward to preparations for the next Christmas – 1954. All wards had a series of small rooms. Kitchen, sterilising room, nurses cloak room, linen cupboard, bathroom, sluice. The latter was the home of the bedpans, dirty laundry, floor cleaning buckets, etc. They usually had a large porcelain draining board and were relatively spacious, and even the wildest imagination would hardly see them as romantic settings. However...

Mayfair One was the main private patients' ward, where, with one exception of two beds, all the patients were in single rooms. Sister was splendid. Yet another of the thirty-year brigade, she was calm, kind, slow-moving but aware and astute. She even talked to her nurses!

I remember her reminiscing about Lord Nuffield – William Morris, the car manufacturer – 'sitting at that table, THERE, and writing a cheque for £40,000'. That cheque was far from his only donation. Shortly before my set left, in 1955, the Wingfield Morris Orthopaedic Hospital was renamed the Nuffield Orthopaedic Centre.

Anyway, back to Christmas preparations. Each patient on Mayfair One was to have a 'Christmas tree', which was actually a small pot of white painted twigs. I, along with John – a medical student and son of the nurses' GP, who was working as a hospital porter in his vacation, which undergraduates did quite often – was sent to the sluice to paint the twigs with ceiling white.

Result! We had never met before but the attraction was immediate. Instinctively we kept our friendship secret, horrified at the thought of hospital gossip, although at home I spent hours talking to my mother about him. At work, having invited me to go to the cinema, to see *The Robe*, we had difficulty finding a private moment in which to arrange a meeting.

After he returned to London he wrote wonderful letters which I kept for decades. We met once, for a country walk when he was home for the weekend, but soon after that came the final letter. He had fallen in love with someone else.

Luckily it arrived when I had a morning off and had taken it up on to the flat roof of the nurses' home to read. Back on duty staff nurse asked if I was all right. It must have been obvious that I had been crying – for ages – but I assured her I was OK.

Patients need cheerful nurses, not woeful ones, and private problems must be left outside the ward doors.

Mayfair had a fascinating crowd of patients, including an impecunious retired army major whose friends used to send him food hampers from Fortnum and Mason. One morning he told me to go and make a slice of toast; when I took it to him he put a spoonful of caviar on and said I might never get another chance to try it. Although I did like it, the pate de foie gras he gave some of us on another occasion was much more to my taste. Delicious! (Though it went off my list of favourites when I learnt of the cruelty involved in producing it.)

An even more generous patient was one of the world's millionaires. Baron von Rothschild. Why 'von' is a mystery; years later I was able to confirm exactly which member of the famous family he was, though no 'von'. Flat in bed with a back problem, he was in for a fortnight, with traction to both legs.

He liked Julie, a sophisticated and sparky girl in my set, and when he learnt that it was her birthday he asked what she would like as a present from Paris. She asked for French gloves and they arrived next day. This caused such a sensation that he called each of us to see him and asked the same question. Unable to think, rather doubtfully, I asked for pearls, thinking of good artificial ones. Before I could explain he demurred and suggested costume jewellery, which struck me as a much better idea. The following afternoon he gave me a box several inches square.

Dark red cardboard with gold CD letters all over, inside was a heavy necklace. Three rows of irregular pearly blue/grey beads, about the size of hazelnuts, with between each bead a circlet of six rhinestones. These were set between two facets of gold metal. Every bead/circlet unit was jointed to the next loop with a twist of fine gold wire. On one end of the linked strands was a large hook identical to those in hook and eye fastenings, but there was no eye on either end, only three smaller beads hanging downwards. I had opened the box in the ward office. Like me, everyone was enchanted – but no one could work out where the hook was to go. The down-hanging length looked too fragile and anyway would unbalance the whole. Not that balance, or any other trial, was feasible over uniform.

Reluctantly, I crept back to the Baron's room to ask the advice of his mistress. The situation was that his wife, a plump, undistinguished looking hausfrau, mother of his three children, visited every morning. For the rest of the day Mrs Churchill kept him company. She was a hard, glamorous, sophisticate, who used to pop grapes into his mouth with her scarlet taloned fingers. She was not friendly. More about her in a minute, meantime I explained the dilemma.

With a pitying expression she demonstrated that the hook did in fact fit the chain, allowing adjustment to three different lengths. Then sneeringly, she asked if I knew what the letters CD on the box stood for. Of course I had to admit that I did not. 'Christian Dior' said she.

This tale of the necklace has been told often and is still vivid in my memory. The beads have been worn and admired innumerable times and now, seventy years later, I still love them. Some years into their third decade they began to feel their age and some broke off. They were most skilfully reattached by a colleague at the QARANC Training Centre (Queen Alexandra's Royal Army Nursing Corps). She was a theatre sister with a keen interest in jewellery and she mended the necklace with very fine wire, normally used for certain types of suturing in the operating theatre. It was seldom the suture material of choice and she had obtained a packet with difficulty. Giving me the remainder, she warned of rare availability and also that it was fragile, so I would be unwise to wear 'the Baron's beads' too often. They are still intact today.

Mrs Churchill is not. She died in 1997, as Mrs Pamela Harriman, American Ambassador in Paris, described by her second husband proudly as 'the greatest courtesan of the century'. Her long, detailed obituary in the *Telegraph* is absolutely fascinating. Sister on Mayfair One told us that when the Baron left – he discharged himself – he went to stay at Blenheim Palace. His wife and children, and Pamela Churchill and her ex-husband Randolph Churchill, went too.

It was also on Mayfair that I returned from a day off to be told at report: 'There is a perfect man in Room Two for you. He is 6ft 7in tall.' David was only in for two days, having cut a tendon in a finger when climbing *into* college (very uncharacteristic). By the second day he apparently agreed with the staff, and when I went into his room to do the inevitable damp-dusting he asked me to go out with him. I sat under his bed for ages – the complicated metal 'Lawson-Tait' frame (for adjusting the bed at a variety of angles) surely never got such a good dusting in its life, but it was easier than facing him. Refusing his invitation I confided my feelings for John (who hadn't ended our relationship at that point), but David had an instant answer. Surely, even if eventually we should get married, I would want to have other friends as well? So I went to the cinema followed by tea, but felt uncomfortable and refused further meetings.

Several months later – after John's final letter – I needed a partner for a hospital dance, so I contacted David. He was pleased to accept my invitation. We went out together for the next four years, having a great deal in common and each encouraged by our families. My mother and little sister Jenny adored him, and David was very fond of my mother. Jenny, aged 8, told him to marry her if I refused and apparently, when she met him decades later, told him off for not doing so, though she was by then happily married herself, with three children. It was no good, I could not, did not, have the slightest feeling for him.

He kept in touch with my mother for many years and when she died both Jenny and I said we must let David know. Years after that, when driving in an unfamiliar part of the country, I realised I was near the school where David was a successful, hugely liked and respected headmaster. It was a happy meeting and he took me home to meet his wife. I enjoyed telling him a story of how much he had impressed the father of one of his pupils

The story arose at the Queen Alexandra's Training Centre, where I was doing a course, in 1976 or '77 which included, for the first time ever, two male RAMC nursing officers – shock, horror! One of them, Alan, was called away to his son's boarding school; the lad had sustained a head injury while climbing in his dormitory. Telling us all about it on his return, Alan was full of praise for the way the headmaster had dealt with the situation and for the kindness and care he and his wife had received. It became clear that it was David's school, a rare local authority Grammar School with some boarders. When the tale was finished I remarked that I had spent four years telling that headmaster that I would not marry him. Not strictly accurate but near enough and the effect was all I hoped for. (I omitted this part from my retelling of the tale to David.) As far as the QAs were concerned I was a middle-aged spinster who had never had a boyfriend nor even looked for one, so it was doubly satisfying.

It is always fun to shock people. At one of the dances in the hospital gym – I cannot remember if David was my partner – I remember losing my balance and sliding to the floor, right in front of matron, who gave me an icy look. No doubt she thought I had been indulging in the gin or similar, though none was officially available. Needless to say I had not, it was just my two left feet being more awkward than usual. The sum of my memories of matron are pretty dreadful.

Early in my training I was ill for a few days, an odd episode which included paralysed arms during one night. Matron told my mother she would never have accepted me had she realised that I would not take care of my health – a remark that mystified both my mother and me. Could it have been a stock comment when she was irritated by concerned parents? Later in my training she told me that my parents were a great handicap to me, for which I never forgave her – though it was my dear father who had provoked it. Having arranged to give me a lift to the dentist, he turned up at the Nurses' Home at 10 am instead of 10.30 am so of course I was not there. He went up to Matron's office to ask where I was! It was a thermometer though which provoked her to real fury.

All broken thermometers meant a visit to matron. Surprisingly, she was forgiving when I took in a dozen. Nasty blip in my first night duty. Perhaps less surprisingly, when I took just one thermometer not all that long afterwards, she was extremely angry. By then I was well into my senior year and though not given to breaking things was still all too frequently inept. She gave me the option of leaving then and there, or having six weeks in which to improve. Having opted for the six weeks, I waited at the end of them with trepidation, for the summons to Matron's office. It never came. The lack of follow up still angers me on the rare occasions when remembering it.

(April 2005. Imagine my utter astonishment this morning, finding in my 1955 diary, a comment I have never remembered. My father had written to me saying that matron had told Mr Markby, the hospital chaplain and our vicar, that I was one of the best! How odd.

What I have always remembered is that at the time of the six week worry he preached a sermon at Evensong which I recognised was for my benefit. It must be admitted that I did not understand it very well, but it was cheering nonetheless.)

The remaining weeks flew but a last minute blow was in store. Before our final exams we were to have a week's study block, revising in the school of nursing. Much of Orthopaedics I had always found hard to understand, but the senior tutor, Sister Stone (later Matron) was a genius at making things clear. She lectured my set all too rarely but was to take our revision block. My set was divided into three, and my group was to do the first week. Three days before, we were told that Sister Stone had to be away next week unexpectedly, but our group was bright enough to manage working on our own. I passed hospital finals with one mark. In National Finals for the Orthopaedic Nursing Certificate I was 158 out of how many? Possibly 200.

On 29 October 1955 I did State Practical and Oral exams in the morning, went to David's degree ceremony in the Sheldonian Theatre at 2 pm, travelled to London next day with his parents and sister – and then was on my own. I stood at a bus stop just south of Waterloo Bridge, on a cold, murky, miserable evening, in bleak surroundings, wondering what lay ahead. Before leaving Wingfield reminisces for good, I suddenly remembered my breast lump which, though it occurred while I was at the Wingfield, had useful outcomes both at King's and later in life. One night about three months before finals I found a lump in my left breast while getting ready for bed. My diary just says 'didn't like it'. Actually I had a sleepless night mostly thinking about dying. By the time I saw the nurses' doctor, who was also my family one, next morning, I was sure the lump was benign. Thanks to a lecture just the week before, all at once I recalled being told that benign tumours were encapsulated. Since mine felt clearly defined, much like a golf ball, thoughts of dying were instantly switched off.

That lecture was remarkably fortuitous as it was the only 'general' one we had in two years, as opposed to Orthopaedics. A Registrar talked to us, chiefly about types of cancer, and of course the timing was ideal.

Having the lump removed was a most useful experience. All doctors and nurses – indeed, all hospital staff – should undergo surgery. For me it was interesting to be a patient in a general hospital ward at the Radcliffe Infirmary, to have an anaesthetic and, memorably, to use a bedpan. From the privileged 'First on the List' position, I was ignominiously sent to the bottom of it after a misunderstanding led to me being given lunch. So instead of theatre at 2 pm it was past 6 pm, but at least that allowed me to join in a ward service. Despite having had my pre-med, I was able to sing a hymn at the top of my voice and enjoyed doing it.

The thing about the anaesthetic was realising afterwards that, rather than merely sleeping in my bed, all sorts of things had happened to ones' person. Very strange. As for the bedpan, staff nurse asked me to use one as soon as I began to wake up.

In those days anaesthetics were less refined and their effect on smooth muscle was liable to provoke retention of urine, so ensuring post-op micturition was an important part of care. Obediently I lifted up my rear to have the bedpan put in place. To my astonishment I was told to lift my bottom up, and I felt half way to the ceiling before, it seemed, there was room for it. Many times in the following years I was able to sympathise with people feeling the same. Even though I was only in the ward two and a half days I did not escape the wrath of Sister. No – that is an exaggeration; but because I had been vomiting all morning she looked at me with disdain when serving lunches. 'And I don't suppose you want any?' said she. Quite right, though I did not feel too bad. It was another common post-op problem in those days. The only fear I had was of pain, but there was never more than slight discomfort.Due to vomiting I was not discharged the following afternoon, but the morning after that. In fine fettle I went home to meet my 16 year old cousin who was up from Somerset on a visit. It transpired that she had never been to the theatre except to see a pantomime, so that needed to be remedied at once. *South Pacific* was on at the New Theatre, so I phoned to book seats for that evening. We loved it, and afterwards I took her to her first ever coffee bar – in 1954 Oxford was said to have the first coffee bar in the country. I remember it well – all spindly legged 1950s' chairs and laminated tables. There I asked for a cappuccino only to have my showing off fall flat when the waitress asked 'What's that?'

The next day I stayed in bed all day. Telling my mother I felt all right was perfectly true, except that I had no energy, a sort of vague lassitude. And that was another incredibly useful experience because times without number I have warned people they may have something similar happen, or explained that it is common; a good post-op day followed by a poor one, but there is no need to worry. Patients just feel reassured if it has happened to nurses.

A couple of decades later while in Nepal, a colleague – not a nurse – much older than I had been, found a lump. She found it hard to accept, though told it was surely a fibrous adenoma. Much commoner, in fact surprisingly common, in younger women. I was so pleased to take her to my room and show her the scar, for it did the trick and she was hugely cheered. Perhaps most helpful of all though, has been that from the night I discovered that lump until now, I have not been afraid of death.

At King's I met with death for the first time and was not daunted. It is sad when someone – anyone – dies alone, even if they are unconscious. Some nurses find it difficult to stay with the dying, but thanks to the night of lump discovery, together with my Christian beliefs, I have been given the strength to cope with saying goodbye. At King's no one even referred to laying out. It was called the Last Washing, and when all was ready Sister came in to say a prayer before we began.

Having long wanted to do my general training at St Thomas's, where my aunt trained and my father had been a patient, it became easy to change my mind. Staff nurses at the Wingfield were nurses who had done their general training first and were now doing a one year post-registration orthopaedic course. With few exceptions they had qualified in one of the London hospitals, so that we students heard tales about all of them. For reasons I cannot remember St Thomas's began to seem rather unappealing, whereas King's sounded reasonable. Three of my friends intended going there too, whereas the confident lass from Randle days was transferring to St Thomas's. We met up there once after we had qualified. I was fascinated to find that it felt more like King's than any other hospital I had been in. Everyone at King's used to refer to it as the 'little cottage hospital down by the river'.

Matron interviewed each of us about our future intentions. Not knowing my ideas, she said she knew something of each of the London teaching hospitals, and then recommended King's which she thought would suit me. I was happy to agree. The day in London for my interview was more important for seeing John than anything to do with training.

Chapter 2

King's College Hospital London SE5

1955–1959

THREE YEARS AT King's began on 30 October 1955. The bus from Waterloo Bridge took me to Denmark Hill, opposite the hospital, via the Elephant and Castle. The elephantine Dept. of Health brutalist block had not been built, nor indeed few other new buildings.

Ten years after the end of the war London was still drab, dreary and barely rebuilt anywhere, though the Festival Hall was glossy and fresh, a permanent legacy of the Festival of Britain. Walking past the Festival Hall en route to Hungerford Bridge and central London was a frequent choice. One day I went in to the hall to see a widely praised exhibition of photographs entitled 'The Family of Man'. I thought it absolutely marvellous and regretted that the excellent catalogue was well beyond my means. Ten years later, browsing in a bookshop in San Francisco, suddenly there in front of me was The Family of Man. Easily affordable, exhibited with joy when I returned to the ship, and still treasured.

The Nurses Entrance was at the Denmark Hill end of the main façade of the hospital. Inside was a small room like a college porter's lodge, where someone was always on duty until late evening. Staff were welcomed, messages taken and post handed out, lost property retained etc. Complementary theatre tickets were frequently available there.

I was soon reunited with the other three from the Wingfield – which had been renamed the Nuffield Orthopaedic Centre just before we left. A big meeting had been called to tell all the staff about the change. Lord Nuffield who, as William Morris, had founded Morris Motors car factory, was interested in medical matters and had donated so many sums of money it was felt an appropriate way to reflect and thank him for his generosity. In earlier days at the Wingfield one or two discreet hints had been dropped that he was *too* interested. Doctors do hate being questioned by lay-people, particularly those who have their own ideas. They did in those days anyway. However, he was eventually given credit for a vast improvement in anaesthetics, not least by endowing a Chair of Anaesthetics in the University. He had suffered at least one bad experience with anaesthetic when young.

At King's our official welcome was from the Second Deputy Matron, Sister Kerr-Smith, a lovely woman who was friendly and approachable. For affiliated nurses like us – others might have done children's nursing or TB for example – it was felt wise that we gained a few weeks' ward experience before going into second year study block. Each of us was told which ward we were to report to in the morning and I could not have been less surprised when told 'Lister'.

King's had originally been a Christian foundation staffed by nuns. For this reason Matron was always known as Sister Matron and the ward Sisters by their Christian names. Sister Lilian of Lister was renowned. Her fearsome reputation was recounted by more than one staff nurse at the Wingfield and I had known of her for months. For almost as long, I had 'known' that Lister would be my first ward. Premonition, 'second sight', call it what you will – foreknowing can be a mixed blessing. Apparently my Highland grandmother certainly said so. She was known to have 'the sight', a fact I had known of since childhood, but what a shock when decades later a cousin showed me a crystal ball which had belonged to her. My own premonitions are rare and often of little moment, but always I try to disregard them. It does not stop the quiet conviction one feels.

After all that, my first day on the ward was of so little consequence I cannot remember a thing about it. It later transpired that Sister Lilian was said to like affiliated nurses. She reinforced my ideas about liking to find out for myself for, amazingly, this tall, thin ram-rod straight woman with the severe expression seemed to find me at least no worse than anyone else. She even made a personal remark once, confiding that she found chest surgery, then in its infancy, particularly interesting. Once, I sensed her approval though she never said a word.

It was a memorable episode in any case. Lister was a woman's surgical ward, and although most of our patients came from local areas often a few had some from further afield. One came from Devon, a shy, nervy, elderly spinster who for six years had endured great pain and misery with Crohn's Disease. To combat this nasty problem she was to have a colostomy. A what? It was shocking to learn that it was an exit from the intestines fashioned in the abdominal wall.

Quite apart from far less fuss and publicity about health, no one in those buttoned-up days would have dreamt of talking about such a thing. Even today, though quite widely known, it is hardly a popular topic of conversation. I was soon to become closely acquainted with one.

Careful pre-op preparation was intended to ensure action-free bowel movements for several days post-op, to help the healing process. However, the morning after the operation I returned from coffee to be called by a worried Miss A. Her colostomy, nowadays usually referred to as a stoma, had worked.

I cleaned it up. It worked again. I cleaned it up. It worked a third time. I cleaned it up. This went on and on, the leaking always starting just as I had finished cleaning. At one point Sister Lilian put her head round the screens, said nothing but sent another nurse to help me. Still it worked. Eventually I got the giggles. Then the other nurse got the giggles. Even poor Miss A eventually saw the funny side. An hour and a half after the saga began, it stopped.

I know it was and hour and a half because I did nothing else between returning from coffee and going to lunch. After that it settled down for days, Miss A made an excellent recovery and I have recounted the tale to various patients ever since. It seems to cheer them that a colostomy of all things can induce fits of giggles, and, as the *Reader's Digest* has it 'Laughter is the Best Medicine'. Laughing in the kitchen, however, was not on the menu when, every evening before going off duty, the teaspoons had to be counted. Twenty-four required.

Mentioning coffee reminds me that we could always have dripping on toast at coffee time. There were large bowls of beef dripping on the tables in the nurses' dining room and we made our own fresh toast. The bowls had jellied gravy at the bottom and the whole was utterly delicious. Telling of toast reminds me that when on night duty we often used to make tea, toast or other snacks for the junior housemen. They were all too frequently in the wards until the early hours, trying to catch up with writing patients' notes and battling exhaustion at the same time.

I used to be incensed on their behalf but it was said that their bosses, the consultants, always claimed that they had done so, that it was the way to learn, and to get on with it.

A hilarious story was told to me by a memorable patient indeed – a very senior nurse who was not only an excellent patient but had a great sense of fun too. She was Night Superintendent in a big hospital several miles away and she was doing her rounds one night when she went into a ward kitchen. A doctor had been sitting on a breadbin eating bacon and eggs but she frightened him and he tried to jump to his feet … crash. She found him wedged in the bread bin with his legs in the air and the plate held aloft.

A happier outcome was a bit of a birthday party I decided to have when on night duty on PP1, the main private patients ward. All the consultants could have patients there so visits from several housemen were common. In 1958 there was a glut of strawberries, so I went down to Camberwell Green, able to afford three punnets of strawberries, and some cream and cakes. When I went on duty a normally fierce female patient announced that her secretary had brought strawberries up from the country for me. Then, lo and behold, a dear, elderly doctor told me with delight he had some real Devonshire cream for me! The strawberries almost filled a one gallon jug and we had at least a pint of cream. Five doctors reacted like schoolboys when they saw what was on offer and with three nurses a good time was had by all. We had a particularly amusing and successful game of Consequences, which involved the Min, (Sister Matron) and a senior consultant. One of the boys had never heard of this game before, and at 2 am was sitting in a corner of the office playing it by himself. He wouldn't tell us what nonsense he was concocting.

Unbelievably, the Min – why that nickname? – was a patient in the ward that night. She was admitted as an emergency a couple of days earlier, the only reason she was in King's. It was an unwritten convention that Matrons were never patients in their own hospitals. The Min was a wonderful patient and very sweet to me. Especially one night when I managed to sweep everything off the top of her locker. She apologised at once saying it was entirely her fault, but it wasn't, it was me being clumsy.

It was during this night duty – three months each year, at King's five nights on, two off – that I spent a few nights on PP2, where private maternity patients stayed. There a titled Lady had her own midwife, Sister Helen Rowe. The Lady was unknown, Sister Rowe was famous. She looked after the Queen (then still Princess Elizabeth) at Buckingham Palace when Prince Charles and Princess Anne were born. Lucky Queen. Sister Rowe was lovely and I was certainly lucky to have several conversations with her.

In those days it was traditional for midwives to have blue, almost royal blue, uniforms in honour of the robes of the Madonna. Sister Rowe's dress was the brightest, almost electric, blue imaginable, and with her snow white hair and enormous veil she looked impressive. She was not fat, but round and comfortable, kind and easy. Did she give me one of her veils? How awful that I cannot be sure. She was about to retire, knew I was going to do midwifery, and I do have an enormous, very fine muslin veil which was undoubtedly a gift, though not recorded in my diary. The memory is faint, but I do remember thinking it unlikely there would even be a chance to use it. In fact, the chance came years later, but the size, plus the fine fabric which did not starch stiffly enough, sent it back into the drawer.

In the 1950s training to become a State Registered Nurse took three years, but most of the major hospitals did not award their own, much coveted, badges until the completion of a fourth year. For 'affiliated' nurses, who had already done things such as orthopaedic or paediatric training, the time was reduced. At King's we did three years instead of four, taking state finals at the end of two years instead of three. This should have meant that I left at the end of October 1958, but by then I had had not one, but two March fractures and did not leave until January 1959.

The first caused amusement but comparatively little inconvenience, as my leg was in plaster while I was in study block, going to lectures in the School of Nursing. My friends Margaret and Jill were particularly amused, because March fractures are little known outside orthopaedic circles and of course plastering is a major orthopaedic treatment. Seeing me in plaster delighted some folk. The oddity was the timing. There is a classic description of March fractures. A man works in an office for fifty weeks of the year – a sedentary job – then goes off to

Territorial Army camp and within forty-eight hours is doing a route march. The unexpected stress causes a fracture in one of the small bones in a toe, and he complains of considerable pain, but gets no sympathy or treatment because nothing shows on X-ray. Several days later when callous has begun to form at the site that does appear on X-ray.

In my case I had been running around the wards for two years, wearing approved shoes, so my spontaneous fractured second metatarsal was a mystery. That was in February 1956. Imagine the same bone, other foot, two years later. This time it happened at home and I became a patient of the Radcliffe Infirmary. The Wingfield Consultants had Clinics there and 'RG', Mr R.G. Taylor, saw me. He was a man of few words and unimpressive demeanour. My mother had been a patient of his when he removed a bunion and speaking rather dubiously about him to one of her nurses, she was reproved with the instant rejoinder 'He is quick, neat and efficient.' Nowadays one is lucky to have a toe even strapped up, but then we had walking plasters for six weeks. However, RG decided to leave mine on for an extra week, astounding me with the remark 'Doctors and nurses are not human Mary' – not only an unexpected, human comment, but he called me MARY. Christian names were NEVER used in those days and of course male patients, in particular, had a lot of fun trying to discover them.

That second fracture was much more troublesome than the first, being painful even when in plaster and the muscles refusing to function properly when the plaster was removed. Five weeks of physiotherapy were added to the seven I had already had at home. Was this frustrating? Not at all, it was grand to be at home for so long. With rare exceptions, off-duty and holidays were more eagerly anticipated than on-duty. It is incredible, but true, that in forty years I was always lucky with them, so never suffered the misery of most colleagues who at some time had had to forego a longed-for event or celebration. Friends' weddings were priorities for many of us and in 1956 I went to tremendous one in Yorkshire. My parents were annoyed, saying that the train fare was far too expensive just for a weekend. In the event it was huge fun from start to finish, a gathering of several friends and memorable for all sorts of reasons. It convinced me that long distance weekends are worthwhile, a theory proved countless times since. It does mean that often I manage as much in a weekend as many people do in a week, and by the same token as much in a week as many do in a fortnight.

A postscript to the Yorkshire wedding was a story which is still amusing. Two of our friends met there with the intention of breaking off their engagement, instead of which it was very much on again by the time they left. The London train from Huddersfield was very crowded, but they wanted a compartment to themselves. They gathered bits of confetti – copious amounts had been showered over all of us – and spread it in the corridor outside the door, with success. The ticket collector arrived to find them sitting in there alone with their arms around each other. But ... one ticket was for London, the other Dover. Peter smiled sweetly at the collector and said 'We are taking our holidays apart this year.'

Reading, knitting and endless letter writing were my main off-duty pastimes at King's, so apart from the need for fewer letters life continued smoothly during the enforced weeks at home. However, evenings off in London sometimes had more interesting things, such a classical record recital, parties with friends, and the monthly meeting of the Listerian Society. Joseph Lister was the Edinburgh surgeon who recognised the need for asepsis and introduced the carbolic spray in his operating theatre. He left Scotland for King's in 1877 and his memory was revered in the hospital. The Listerian Society held meetings in the medial school to which were invited a variety of interesting, not always medical, speakers. The lecture theatre was packed on the evening Evelyn Home came. She was the best known Agony Aunt of the time, having a famous (by today's standards, bland) letters page in *Woman* magazine. After her talk it was fascinating to hear her being quizzed – by the men! Question after question, revealing their in-depth knowledge of her attitudes and answers.

It was about this time someone told me that *Vogue* was one of the magazines subscribed to by the Junior Common Room at Balliol College. Is it still?

Visits to the cinema were quite common, and free tickets for theatres were often available. It was thanks to the free tickets that I saw a side variety of productions, from *Waiting for Godot* to *The King and I*. It must be confessed that I walked out of the former at the interval, but the latter could not have been more exciting. This famous musical was nearing the end of a very long run at Drury Lane and my friend Margaret and I had seats in the front row of the stalls. It was a cold night and the leader of the orchestra came back after the interval rubbing his hands.

We sympathised, then some unknown impulse made me ask him if there were ever any opportunities for back stage visits. To our astonishment he promptly invited us to meet him at the stage door after the show. He gave us a marvellous tour, particularly interesting due to the large number of props used. Each in its designated place and including things like Siamese musical instruments and at least one giant papier mâché animal head. In one corner was a small box-like structure, an almost-on-stage dressing room, for 'Anna Leonowens', played by Deborah Kerr, to do a fast costume change, when there was not enough time for her to go up to her third floor room. It was all unforgettable and of course we were thrilled. In those days nurses were hugely respected and all sorts of people were very kind to us.

Because King's was five miles from the centre of London we did not have to be in until midnight, but woe betide us if five minutes late. The Nurses' Entrance locked; the fierce night porter at the grand Main Entrance taking our names; an interview in Fleet Street next morning – the Admin corridor where Sister Matron, her deputy and two assistants had their offices. For the early hours of Christmas morning we were given an extension until 1.30 am, to enable many of us to go to Midnight Communion on Christmas Eve. Four of us wanted to go to St Martin's-in-the-Fields, but the timetable was a bit tight and I agreed to book a taxi. Across The Strand from the back of St Martin's is Charing Cross Station, so I went to the first taxi in the rank there. The driver laughed at me. Said he might be anywhere in London at that time on that night. 'Oh dear,' said I, 'that's no good. We have to be back at the hospital by 1.30 am.' 'You a nurse?' he asked. 'Yes,' I replied. 'I'll be there.'

After the service we stood on the steps as the crowds disappeared and the others got quite irritated with me as we went on waiting. Suddenly he was there, full of apologies because he had had a fare far out into North London. We were back by 1.30.

Days off in London were nearly always spent shopping or exploring, and I enjoyed many of the most famous places, including listening to a debate in the House of Commons from the Strangers' Gallery; no booking needed, one just walked in via Westminster Hall. One day I went to the Imperial War Museum and was no sooner inside the door than confronted with a familiar scene. A small oil painting was labelled 'A Typical Food Office'.

I knew it well, as a high ceilinged, oddly shaped hall down in St Ebbes's, a poor part of Oxford, having gone there to collect milk and orange juice tokens for my baby sister in the late 1940s.

The surprise was out of all proportion to the size of the painting. Museum exhibits were academic; historical, rare, important – think of the Egyptian mummies and Alfred's Jewel in the Ashmolean, or my favourite pterodactyl in the University Museum. Nothing with the remotest personal connection to me.

The bombing in London had been completely outwith my experience, but the aftermath was still all too evident in the mid-'50s. The great cry was for housing, so the journey from Camberwell into central London was, in places, a procession of hoardings and boarded up, derelict commercial sites. Hoardings did not conceal the huge craters all round St Paul's Cathedral; one had a vast metal tank in it, still full of brackish water, ready for fire fighting. Redevelopment had to wait, commercial buildings were not a priority. In late 1958 my room in the Nurses' Home was on 'Fourth North', the highest floor. The view was spoilt by a tall school building opposite, but in the distance it was possible to see three much taller buildings. I thought I could count twenty storeys. How thrilling! Especially if one could live on one of the top floors. They must have been some of the earliest tower blocks of flats and to me they were exciting. Whether any of my friends agreed I cannot remember, and perhaps they were unaware, as by then most of them lived out in rented flats. Economic madness to me. Perhaps I was always a bit of a loner, having been encouraged from the age of 12 to do things on my own if friends were not free.

With the constraints of off-duty rotas, lone expeditions were quite common, so I learnt at an early age that people talk more readily to one person than a couple. Mercifully my parents never told me that I should not talk to strangers, for which I have been grateful all my life. Gleefully, it must be admitted, passing this wisdom on to parents and grandparents who want to wrap their precious sprigs in the proverbial cotton wool.

Very different from climbing the dome of St Paul's or exploring London Zoo was an expedition one summer evening in South London. When in study blocks, or on night duty, we went to live in Hambledon House, on the edge of Dulwich golf course, on the far side of charming Dulwich Village. Three of us went for a walk up towards Sydenham, and we found a derelict railway tunnel. Maybe someone had told us about it, certainly we knew the line went to Crystal Palace and also that the tunnel was half a mile long. Or was it a quarter? Anyway we braved it, though maybe only because we could see a pinpoint of light at the far end. Though glad to be able to say we had done it – in both directions – it was agreed not necessary to recommend to our friends. Too dull. My main memory is of unexpected drops of very cold water landing on my head and bare arms. Luckily not many, as the tunnel was basically dry.

David came up one year for the Boat Race – I still have the Race favour of wooden crossed oars, with blade ends and a ribbon bow of Oxford blue – and afterwards (Cambridge won) we went to the Ideal Homes Exhibition. There we acquired some food samples, including cheese, and decided to use these for a picnic next day. Unable to decide where to eat it we agreed to meet next day under the clock at Victoria station.

We had our picnic on Beachy Head. Quite why we two penniless students rejected all the London parks is forgotten, but the day is not. From Eastbourne we caught a bus to Pevensey, walked round the castle ruins and then had tea in a small tearoom in Pevensey Bay. There were small antiques for sale and David bought me an oval, tortoiseshell hand mirror which I used for years, until it began to fall apart (not thrown away though). Back at Eastbourne Station we were shocked to find our train was a Pullman and we had to pay extra. No option, David had to get back to Oxford and any later trains were too late. It was way beyond our normal expeditions, and so was, even more, New College Commemoration Ball.

Like the Summer Balls in Cambridge they are formal, glamorous and last all night, with a variety of bands and cabarets.. There are a few each year, but no college has them annually.

David was a Brasenose man now doing a DPhil (in low temperature physics) and he told me he had been invited to join a party for the ball at New College but it was too expensive. A double ticket was six guineas. At my insistence we always split expenses in half, but in addition to his share of the ticket David would have to acquire a dinner jacket. We walked in silence down The High as David wrestled with my anxiety to accept. Outside the Examination Schools he stopped abruptly, turned to me and said 'We'll go.' My mother made my dress, which was worn for years, always loved. Last seen on stage sixty years later, worn by a 'Princess' in a local village amateur dramatic pantomime.

At the Royal Eye Hospital, nearer Victoria than King's, I was on duty all day but allowed to leave early in time to catch a coach home. The ball started at 9 pm but there was to be a dinner party for our group, in college, beforehand. It was agreed that we would have to miss that as I would not be home in time. Hence, as I got ready, my mother made me a hearty pile of sandwiches and, would you believe, a cup of cocoa, as in those days I still rarely liked coffee.

We arrived at New College to discover ten people and a butler awaiting our arrival. Somehow I found space for a cold, but substantial, three course meal. After that we were shown to our rooms, that is a sitting room and bedroom just for us two; there was the same for each couple. The undergraduates had gone down so although there was furniture in situ it all looked bare and forlorn, but in any case we were quite shocked. In the early hours we went back to these rooms but immediately realised it would be fateful to sit down, if we did we wouldn't keep going until the end of the ball at 6 am. With difficulty David had persuaded a florist to make a corsage of white rose buds. She told him they did not last and bruised easily, but they were lovely when he gave them to me. Sadly she was right, and they were abandoned in our college rooms.

We danced to Tommy Kinsman and Chris Barber, two of the most famous bands of the day. Tommy Kinsman's band played traditional music whilst Chris Barber played jazz. The Ball included a cabaret featuring Tommy Cooper, complete with fez, then at 3 am we walked to the Oriel College ball to listen to Humphrey Lyttleton play his trumpet. There was a champagne bar at Oriel. Maybe the same in New College. Certainly I had two glasses, other alcohol forgotten, though neither of us ever drank much.

I think there may have been a buffet in hall, and at 6.15 am everyone still present gathered in the quad for a group photograph. After that David and I went punting on the river for a couple of hours and then had breakfast at The Kemp, a favoured undergraduate restaurant in The Broad. We walked back to New College, in a vain hunt for perfume I had left on a shelf in the Ladies, and then to The High to catch a bus home. Walking down The High, and standing at a bus stop in full evening dress at 9 am as everyone else is on their way to school or work, requires a nonchalant attitude…

Talking of alcohol reminds me that nowhere in Oxford was open for lunch on Sundays except perhaps expensive restaurants or hotels. Lunches were available in Hall but I'd heard they were unpopular due to poor food. Anyway, David and five of his friends formed an exclusive Sunday lunch club, to which only two or three special girl friends were invited. Each man took it in turn to choose a different kind of bread, cheese and wine, served in his digs and sampled by the assembled group.

Someone who shared digs with David was Ian Boyd. Not only did he achieve a First, he was also an international athlete. He came sixth in the 1500 metres at the Olympic Games in Melbourne in 1956, and sent me a postcard of a koala bear, postmarked the Olympic Village. It was thoughtful of him but I knew he had only sent it because he thought I was the sort of person who would boast of such a souvenir and show it to all and sundry. He was wrong. Only my parents and David saw it.

Ian and I had met several times, I had been to watch him run at the White City, had been an overnight guest in his home (Olympic rings on my towels) but we were just not on the same wavelength. There was no hostility, just indifference.

Several years later, after Ian had married an occupational therapist and emigrated to New Zealand, and I was living and working in Plymouth, David came to the city for a wedding, and came to see me while there. He confided that, with the distance of time, he could admit that Ian thought 'there wasn't much about me'.

He was dumbfounded when I replied that I already knew that. Men are dense sometimes.

The sad thing is, I knew Ian was right. I do not, and never have had, any compelling interests or abilities. Though I have enjoyed a wide spectrum of superficial ones, and have had an extraordinarily lucky life. Not least with Oxford. It is a wonderful place. As examples, I had a school tour of the Bodleian Library, including the underground bookstacks and conveyor; I sang in a music festival in the Sheldonian Theatre; through the Youth Fellowship, I got to listen to a debate in the Union. By a great piece of good fortune the subject had been changed at the last minute and the motion was That This House Will Never Admit Women. The motion was carried. (My sister, eleven years younger than me, was at Holton Park Girl's Grammar School in the same class as Ann Mallalieu, who became the first female President of the Cambridge Union.)

Saturday shopping trips followed by many wanderings around colleges before going home; Christmas lectures in the University Museum; theatrical productions, large and small, in college gardens; watching Torpids from a college barge; May morning, once before school when a crowd of us fried sausages for breakfast in the Botanical Gardens after following the Morris dancers through the streets, and once, on top of Magdalen Tower itself – amazing. A colleague who, at the last minute, could not be off duty knew I was at home on holiday. She contacted her Magdalen boyfriend and sent him to find me so that the precious opportunity would not be wasted.

Is it any wonder that I feel that I have had the advantage of so many things Oxford has to offer, without ever having to do a shred of study. Incidentally, for years before going to King's I used to say I wanted three years in London to get to know it. My family detested it, so we never went during my childhood, but when living there I loved it, and still do. The only difference is that while knowing it – and knowing my way about it – is a joy, after three years there was never any wish to live there again. Visits yes, always stimulating,

Talking of Ian reminds me of a quite different sporting event in London. There was a Test Match being played at The Oval which even now is famous in the annals of cricket. Two English bowlers, Lock and Laker, were disposing of the Australian wickets with panache, and by the final afternoon the news was full of their exploits.

My mother was quite a keen cricket fan; I was working at the Royal Eye which was in easy walking distance of The Oval, and had an afternoon off. No matter that I would have to wear my outdoor uniform – navy raincoat and beret – which was strictly for travelling between hospitals, residences or going down to Camberwell Green ONLY. Blow the rules. Off I went, and easily got a good seat, though The Oval is large and the players looked small. Cheers. A wicket down. I was looking at a pigeon. Cheers. A second wicket down. I was looking the other way. Cheers. A third wicket gone. I was watching someone in the crowd. I never saw a single wicket fall.

Back at King's – not before time after all these pages of off-duty – at one point I almost fell out of nursing. Having looked forward to a medical ward, Pantia Ralli, male medical, it proved disappointing and difficult. Sister and staff nurses were displeased and I was dispirited, dissatisfied even more than usual with my efforts, and dejected. One evening when phoning home tears began. After that the sequence of events is a blur, though my mother urged me to go home on my next days off, and at some point I had an interview with Sister Matron. She was kind and encouraging. My only precise memory is complaining that it took me half an hour to do a proper blanket bath, teeth, hair, nails, pressure areas etc., which was far too long. To my astonishment the Min sympathised, agreeing with my timing and saying she too had found them a problem!

Our next encounter was when she presented a group of us with our 'bonnets', the caps worn by all the State Registered staff. It was a famous ritual, not least because the Min's words were frequently quoted with glee. 'Bonnets' as fourth year nurses were known, insisted that we would solemnly be told 'you are now inextricably woven into the fabric of the hospital'. Could she really come out with such a dictum? She could and she did and believe me, not a ghost of a smile, let alone a giggle, escaped us.

Hospital exams were in September 1957 and State ones in October. The hospital ones were agreeably easy, including the ever dreaded practical one. There was no pre-packaging in existence, every piece of equipment required for a procedure was stored separately somewhere, and for things like dressings, arranged on trolleys in a series of bowls, kidney dishes and gallipots. Quite apart from exams, lists and notebooks were always forbidden and everything and every patient had to be memorised. For me, a nightmare, not so much the patients but certainly the trolleys. There was also a specific problem with the trolleys. Imagine an array of shiny stainless bowls etc, each covered by its upside down twin. The slightest jolt and slither, crash, disaster,

Consultants used to take our exams, and I was asked to set up a trolley for a blood transfusion. There are, or were, minimum and maximum ways of preparing for a blood transfusion and I had the lot. The examiner took one look at the trolley, with silly upside down bowls and bits in profusion and he exclaimed 'You've got everything there but the kitchen sink', and he did not lift a single lid to see if the right stuff was inside.

State finals were a different kettle of fish. Practicals were taken alternately at King's or at St Giles, Camberwell, the LCC (London County Council) hospital, about a mile away en route to Peckham. It was our turn to go to St Giles, and we had an unpleasant arrival, being greeted by a Sister who sneered at us for coming from King's. We were quite lucky to be there at all, as some 50 per cent of all the hospital staff succumbed to Asian Flu that October. With finals to be taken I 'decided' that I would certainly NOT have Asian Flu. Nor did I, but later missed what promised to be a superb Christmas on the children's ward, due to ordinary flu.

One problem with being an affiliated nurse was fitting in all the specialist areas we needed. My theatre experience was negligible, having spent nine out of ten weeks in the anaesthetic room of the ear, nose and throat theatre. Before the exam I asked my friend Peggy to show me a general set. She had done a lot of time in general theatres and loved it, being a good practical nurse. A general set was the basis for many operations, specialist pieces being added according to whatever operation was to be done. When 'laying up' one always began with knife, fork, spoon i.e. scalpel, forceps and a retractor. Margaret took me through it and in the exam I was asked to lay up for an appendicectomy. That was not too bad, but then I was asked to talk through the operation. Getting down to the appendix was straightforward, but once there I was clueless. Just about to dry up completely, wondering what on earth happened to the wretched thing next, when the tutor thanked me and went on to something else. Presumably I sounded as if I knew.

My specialist experience included three months at the Maudsley, the London Post-Graduate Psychiatric teaching hospital. It was directly opposite King's on the other side of Denmark Hill. Just at the end of my first twelve months people in my set were given the chance to go there if they wished. It was to be counted as part of our training, but only for volunteers.

We were the first King's nurses to go and we spent Christmas 1956 there. My ward was women's acute admission, with twenty-three beds. Violent patients of either sex were admitted to a separate building called The Pavilion, but our patients were the next most acutely disturbed. Sister was surprisingly young, attractive, pleasant, wise and above all, calm. She had been in charge of the ward for three years and was ideal for the job. Both hospital and ward could not have been better for an insight into the care of the mentally ill, because they were at the forefront of modern thinking, with able doctors and tutors and no sign of some of the wilder theories later promulgated. Bedlam, the lunatic asylum of notoriety, was succeeded by the Bethlem Royal Hospital, built in Monk's Park, South Beckenham and part of the Maudsley.

Although our ward doors had to be kept locked the policy in general was already obsolete. We saw this when taken on visits to two of the vast Victorian asylums built in the country beyond – in those days – the outskirts of London. The Maudsley was small, but these hospitals had miles of high ceilinged empty corridors and huge wards which originally housed up to one hundred patients. Overall their capacity, even in the 1950s, was between 2,000 and 2,500 patients. Strenuous efforts were being made to modernise, to make the cavernous wards smaller and everywhere more colourful and comfortable. Needless to say a daunting task given the post-war constraints. I am still glad to have seen them; remain indignant at the way they were vilified, and scandalised at their destruction with no replacements whatever. They sheltered some extremely vulnerable people.

My three months at the Maudsley were enjoyable, full of interest and insight into the treatment of the mentally ill. When I left, Sister told me she was writing my report and it was 'Excellent'. She also confided that she was leaving. I hoped she was about to tell me that she was getting married, but to my surprise she explained that she felt she had given all that she could in mental care and was about to return to Bristol to do district nursing.

Quite soon after these experiences it was rather regrettable to realise I never wanted to do psychiatric nursing again. Hard to analyse why, but possibly due to being impatient. Wanting the patients to do more to help themselves perhaps? It was precisely because they could not that they were admitted of course, so such an attitude would be not good for them, or me. One thing in no doubt is that I always preferred smaller wards and departments. My last few weeks at King's were especially happy, with a fortnight in Medical Out Patients (MOP) and about three weeks in Casualty

Physicians almost invariably have a gentler approach to life and humanity than surgeons and MOP had some happy clinics – enhanced, too, by a bright, pleasant bunch of medical students, 'Firm B'. One episode made a great impression, on the students I suspect as well as on me. Sir Wilfred Sheldon was an eminent paediatrician, one of whose patients had been Princess Anne. A grandmother brought her granddaughter to clinic, a little girl about 6 years old. Granny was humble, shy, overwhelmed. And terrified. Hardly to be wondered at. She was fearful about her granddaughter, scared at seeing the 'great man' and what he might say; and she'd had to walk through a large room to sit in front of him, surrounded by young medical students and with a nurse there too. Dr Sheldon talked to her. He told her what her worries were about the little girl, making it plain he understood and sympathised. With innumerable notes already available, he explained his own thinking about what treatment was needed and what that would involve. The rest of us did not exist. He was a gentleman having a quiet conversation with a lady who needed reassurance and help. Eventually he encouraged her to ask questions, examined the patient with skill and kindness, confirmed his ideas and courteously sent them on their way. Granny was no longer overwhelmed or terrified.

Casualty was a small department, rarely under pressure. An ambulance driver once confided to me that he and his colleagues were selective. Tramps, drunks and other less than salubrious patrons of their transport were taken to St Giles, as not considered suitable for us! When King's was designated a major Accident and Emergency Centre years later, it was many more years before the department was enlarged and organised properly. No wonder it became a scandal which hit the national headlines on several occasions. It was a happy place when I was there, a good department to work in during my last days at King's.

On my final day the Min presented me with my hospital certificate. There were two possible versions. One stated that the recipient had served the hospital 'with Distinction', the other 'with Satisfaction'.

I could not remember whether the Min had personally given me my certificate, or one of her deputies, so I looked back in my diaries. In those days, my diary entries were all too frequently very brief, so I wasn't sure I'd find much there. Imagine my shock when I read that not only had the Min given me my certificate – despite the day being a Sunday – but, and I quote, 'had an excellent report from Casualty sister; Method etc. Excellent.' 'Takes a lot to make Sister D say that, Nurse!' 'Have got "Distinction" on my certificate and been invited back as a 'green-belt' – a Staff Nurse; denoted by their wide green uniform belts.

Forgetting about the Casualty report was nothing compared to reading of the invitation to return as a green-belt! Was it diminished by knowing it was fairly common? Or my own antipathy to the idea? It cannot have seemed much of a feather in my cap at the time or surely it would not have been forgotten?

No doubt it was at least partly due to a general feeling of disappointment with nursing. I was not a dedicated nurse – I had not found my niche, nor had I found a husband.

Pity about the husband. He was supposed to have turned up in Wingfield days, to save me worrying about General training; then at King's, so no need to do Part I Midwifery; ditto prior to Part II … caution rather than common sense had made me apply to do Part I Midwifery, at Queen Charlotte's in Hammersmith, long before it was time to leave King's.

I had nearly a fortnight at home before going there. Holidays were normally spent at home, or in Somerset with grandparents or aunts and uncles.

In 1958 I achieved my ambition to go down the pit – I had first asked my policeman uncle when I was 8 years old. 'When the war is over will you arrange for me to go down the mine?' Being a policeman, I saw him as a man who could achieve this. The family laughed at me, as they did when the request was repeated several years later. Consequently, after going for a walk one summer evening when spending nights off with my grandparents, it took half an hour of hard talking to convince them their legs were not being pulled. Exploring the mine – wearing a treasured white jacket – I was taken to meet the manager. 'Not THE Mr Chapman!' he exclaimed when I told him where I was staying – clearly my grandfather was known and respected well beyond our small family. He had been the Stationmaster at Midsomer Norton and Welton on the GWR line between Frome and Bristol. (A line long gone; closed and subsequently demolished. Sad, as I have innumerable happy memories of it.)

At 2.30 pm next day the mine fireman took me underground for three hours. Gran had found an old pair of dungarees for me to wear and I was given a miner's helmet. The seams of the Somerset coalfield were narrow and at the coalface the men had to bend or work on their knees. Before leaving the mine the miners, all lovely men, welcoming and jolly, made sure my face was blackened. Afterwards I did not endear myself by telling everyone they should pay double for their coal.

Part of my childhood was hearing their boots tramping home at the end of a shift, particularly at about 6.30 am after the night shift. Also, not calling at their cottages at a certain time, when with Gran collecting 'nursing money', because they would be having their bath – in a tin bath in front of the kitchen fire. Pit head baths not built by the 1950s.

The 'nursing money' was a penny or tuppence a week towards nursing care if needed.

'Proper' holidays were too expensive, though I did manage two. In October 1956 Margaret and I had a memorable week in Edinburgh. We had been advised to stay in the YWCA hostel – the accommodation was basic, with narrow beds in flimsily partitioned cubicles. My first purchase in Edinburgh was a towel, as we discovered we had to provide our own. After three days the Warden asked if we were on holiday and was annoyed when we said yes, telling us the hostel was not for holiday makers. However, as we were only there for a week we were allowed to stay, much to our relief. An extraordinary variety of adventures took us far beyond the mandatory first-time-in-Edinburgh explorations of the Castle, Holyrood House and John Knox's house, though we enjoyed those too. We had a day in St Andrews, a delightful little city, and I have loved it ever since. We went by train; too bad the line no longer exists.

A very good day was doing a coach tour of the Trossachs, and another one exploring Dunfermline and the Abbey. In the main street in Dunfermline, , Biddy, a friend from our group at the Wingfield, now an undergraduate at Edinburgh University, who had come to Dunfermline with us,, was hailed by an old friend from her school days and we soon found ourselves having afternoon tea in the Dockyard Superintendents' House in Rosyth. Another afternoon tea came about because I had told a patient in PPI about my forthcoming holiday. Her immediate response had been that we must go to tea with her cousin and she would write to her. On reflection we decided it would be rude not to accept, so I telephoned, and was invited for that afternoon, though I had an awful suspicion our hostess had never heard of us. She had not – but Mrs B's letter arrived just before we did. There was a second post in those days. We could not have received a warmer welcome in a delightful drawing room in Morningside. We were both impressed by a big cosy fire, not to mention a generous spread of food, and thoroughly enjoyed our visit. An added bonus was our glee at the thought of PPI's Sister's face had she known. Not a bad sort really but she was a notorious snob and if she had been aware that her 'ordinary' patient had titled connections ... our charming hostess was Lady Clows! Not a name I have ever heard of since – hardly surprising as it was forgotten until I wondered if it was in my diary. Too many names have not been recorded.

It was thanks to Biddy that we went to a university lecture on political economy. Biddy did her orthopaedic training with us. I remember her vividly on our first day because I thought she looked the oldest in the group but turned out to be the youngest. She had a thin, rather pale face with a mature expression and mousey/sandy hair, scraped back into a small bun. We never worked together but by all accounts she was a very good nurse, which was easy to believe. Her grandmother had died and left her a legacy, which she decided to spend on going to university and then becoming a teacher. She was a particular friend of Peggy and good fun, so its was grand spending time with her. She wanted to take us to the Student's Union for coffee but decided to smuggle us into a lecture first. We followed her into a large, high, circular auditorium and sat down without being challenged. The place was packed so two extra were hardly noticeable. I thought it would be tactful to look as if I was making notes, so Biddy gave me a piece of thin paper torn from a book of ORDER ONLY forms.

By the end of the lecture I had begged two more pages. To my astonishment I could understand what we were being told and found it interesting. Inflation and deflation were explained; going off the Gold Standard in 1929; exchange rates; boom and bust; all sorts of dull financial things made clear in an easy to understand way. He must have been a brilliant lecturer. Sadly no record of his name, but I do still have my notes. No handouts in those days. Ever since, Edinburgh University has ranked almost a high as Oxford in my affections and I have a soft spot for St Andrew's too. After the lecture we had coffee in the Union as Biddy had planned, then we left her and went off on yet another memorable expedition – J.K. Rowling eat your heart out. We got there first. Roslin Chapel was famous long before Harry Potter and we were keen to see the Prentice Pillar. Even then the chapel was undergoing repairs and I was very impressed by Margaret when she had a long technical discussion with one of the workmen about the details of what he was doing. The chapel was, and is, fantastic. A final memory. Princes Street went on for ever. It still does – after all, it is a mile long.

My other holiday away was eleven days spent on my own exploring Cornwall. By October 1958 the rest of my set had left or were about to, so it was go alone or not at all. For years I had longed to travel on the Cornish Riviera Express, the 10.30 Limited as it was known by the GWR (Great Western Railway) – Grandad's railway. Long after his death I read that it was also known as God's Wonderful Railway, something he would not have approved of, despite his great sense of fun.

From Paddington to Penzance, with a pre-war booklet 'Through the Window', to help identify sights, was exciting, but on arrival I stood on the platform at 5 pm feeling dejected and stupid. It was a grey, dreary evening, I was more than 200 miles from home, knew no one and had nowhere to stay. After this inauspicious beginning I had a wonderful time, but despite seeing innumerable beautiful places and having endless friendly encounters with local people, it was the week in Edinburgh which left the most lasting impressions. My Cornish holiday was probably thought affordable because earlier that month I received three months' additional back pay. It was £3.00. Our salaries varied little throughout our years at the Wingfield and King's, somewhere around £8.00 per month, a little more in our last year after we qualified. Quite recently I heard someone on the radio talking about nursing in the 1950s, or rather, a reference to nurses pay. She was implying shock at our £8.00 per week, so her reaction to the correct amount per month is easy to imagine. We were still getting free board, lodging and laundry, but the majority of girls were increasingly anxious to escape Nurses' Homes and live 'out', in rented flats, though no rebate system existed. Economic nonsense, I thought, nor did I feel restricted by living in. Stodgy, may be? When I started nursing my mother gave me two 'Emergency' pounds to keep in my writing case. They stayed there until after midwifery training when I returned to London and shared a flat with two friends. Then the two notes were in constant use to subsidise me. It was only later I realised how much help my flatmates were getting from their parents.

My parents had very little money, but my mother was brilliant at stretching pounds and she always coped. Eventually the £2.00 was put back in the writing case and stayed there for years. Not quite until £1 bank notes were discontinued, but more of the realisation that finances were much easier and the 'emergency pounds' were no longer needed.

Chapter 3

Queen Charlotte's Maternity Hospital, Hammersmith

1959

NURSES WERE ALWAYS encouraged to go elsewhere after qualifying, to broaden their experience in different hospitals. Midwifery was considered a useful additional qualification and Part I in particular, regarded as almost mandatory for senior posts. It was by far the most common next step, six months in a midwifery training school. Part II required a second six months, necessary to become a State Certified Midwife and actually practice midwifery.

My own reason for doing Part I was a feeling that babies might arrive unexpectedly anywhere at any time. Where this theory came from, not 'evidence-based' in today's jargon, is unknown, but it seemed wise to have some knowledge about what to do in such an emergency. Also, I had never seen a baby born, an event I was keen to watch and training seemed the only way.

Queen Charlotte's was regarded as the premier training school and most anxious applicants stated their intention to continue to Part II, fearing rejection otherwise. Later, after acceptance, I learnt that my 'Part I only' was appreciated by the hierarchy. The irony was, I went on to Part II after all, as many girls did not.

At Queen Charlotte's new pupils joined the training school every month, and many sets were disgruntled, resenting being junior students again after the giddy heights of being State Registered.

The February 1959 group could not have been more different. Several girls had come from hospitals in Northeast England, and two from Scotland, all intent on sampling life in London. They meant to enjoy themselves and, thanks to a couple of lively leaders, we all had a lot of fun.

Training was demanding. We had a heavy schedule of mandatory lectures so that quite often we had to attend one on days off, and even after coming off night duty. Fifty palpations were required – examinations of pregnant tummies – also often necessary during off-duty. Some Consultants gave lectures and, most frequently, a senior Registrar. An arrogant man, he redeemed himself by admitting that twice in the past year he had failed to diagnose twins – before that he would have said such a failure was a disgrace. No scans in those days. He also proved himself gifted at difficult deliveries, so we forgave him his arrogance. If having my own baby, I would have chosen him for my care above any other obstetrician.

The summer of 1959 was one of the hottest of the twentieth century. Tennis was popular and we played on two courts overlooked by all the post-natal wards. One evening I went back on duty to be told by a patient: 'I am so glad you are a better nurse that a tennis player.' Another two patients I remember were both in the private ward. One was an older mum who had sons of 13 and 15, so this baby was a surprise and was to be delivered by an elective Caesarean Section one Sunday morning. One son was to be confirmed that day, in his school chapel, and his father was to be with him but would telephone to confirm the baby's safe arrival. There was great excitement about this at their school because the baby's name was then to be put on the entry waiting list, the first time this had happened actually on the day of birth. It was a boys' only school but there had only been boys in this family for 149 years, so no problem. Except that the baby was a girl. Family thrilled.

Another mum was a member of the Lyons family of tea and Corner Houses fame. She had twins, and so many flowers that despite being in a large room they were lined up in the corridor outside. In with her was a very clever arrangement acknowledging the family being keenly involved in horse racing. The oblong base was a turf race course, with one horse at the finishing post with the name of the first twin on the saddle and the second close behind with the name of the second twin.

I cannot remember details of how it was made except that the horses were wire models covered with carnation petals. I happened to be in the room when her Consultant came to see her. He took one look at the race course, said it was wrong, picked up the second horse and turned it round, bottom towards the winning post. The second twin had been a breech.

Presents for nurses were frequent and generous, not just from wealthy private patients. Boxes of chocolates were common in many wards but sometimes we were given more individual gifts. The most personal one I ever had was astonishing. Given 'from Emily', the baby, her mother told me with pride that it had been chosen by her husband.

He was known and admired for an unusual talent – identifying perfumes to fit personalities. He was happy with his choice for me. So was I! Pierre Balmains' *Joli Madame*. Always my favourite, to my sorrow it was discontinued many years ago, but not before I was able to afford to buy more on two occasions, thanks to duty-free Hong Kong.

As at King's, complementary theatre tickets were often available, but not for the brand new Mermaid Theatre at Puddle Dock in the City. Several of us wanted to go to the first production there, *Lock up your Daughters*. On a glorious summer evening I went off to get tickets for us and then decided to wander round the empty city streets. In Printing House Square, I was looking at photos in *The Times* display window when a foreign girl asked me 'How to get into *The Times*?' We went off to find out and I was told I could go round myself if I went one evening next week. Next I found the Apothecaries hall, then the Guildhall, where a man on duty at the door made some pleasant remark and invited me in. There had been a big function and much clearing up was going on behind the scenes. In the main hall the lights were switched on for me, I was shown the Ambulatory used for receptions, and the servery, then taken on to the dais to sit in the Lord Mayor's chair! There were traditional herbs scattered on the floor and I could smell them. Wonderful evening.

So was the visit to *The Times* the following week. Every evening a group was shown around the printing works, the tour ending with beer and sandwiches in the Board Room. Too bad about the beer, have never liked it, but the tour was engrossing. We watched the highly skilled compositors fitting upside down and backward letters and figures, each a tiny fragment of metal, into slide holders which would be fixed into trays the size of a page. We were forbidden to speak to them as they concentrated. At the time I was oblivious to the fact that these men were some of the most highly paid in the country. Nor did I appreciate that they were led, in their 'chapels', to strike at the drop of a hat and bring newspaper production to a standstill. Nor did I know then, and maybe in 1959 neither did they, that in a few years time their expertise and intransigence would be history. The next part of the tour took us through a major industrial site. The heat and noise were indescribable as we were shown the metal foundry and huge printing presses, the latter spewing out papers at a great rate. These were bundled up and rushed out to vans waiting to drive to the mainline railway stations. The first editions were destined for overnight journeys to the far north and west. Up in the boardroom we were given mementos of our visit, including a copy of the next day's paper, a miniature Air Mail edition, and two booklets about printing and publishing. Best of all we were given our names on a small metal bar in *The Times* capital letters font. The boardroom in the 'Private House' was impressive, with dark panelled walls and a huge shiny table. Maddeningly, I have no memory of other parts of the visit. My diary records that three of us were shown Sir John Walter's private office (who he?), and a dining room. Also the Foreign News Room, where hung a prayer, 'O Lord, help me to keep my big mouth shut until I know what I am talking about.'

It was sad when *The Times* left its historic home in Printing House Square but I felt so glad and privileged to have been there. Several years later I visited the Old Gaol in Abingdon – no longer inhabited by old lags, it was a brand new arts centre. Provincial newspapers had been in the forefront of using new technology and the *Oxford Times* had an exhibition there. What a contrast. Reports were typed directly into small, clean, quiet machines. Production used photographic techniques and far less manpower was necessary. Wapping and the riots were still to come and they had been preceded by a year long strike at *The Times*; such sad ends to proud traditions.

One day I answered a ward phone to a call from *The Times*. Would I confirm that Margaret Elizabeth MacDonald had had a baby yesterday? I think that was the name – certainly all three names had several syllables. No I would not, I would transfer the call to Sister. As a lowly junior pupil I was wary because TWO Margaret Elizabeth MacDonalds had been delivered within hours of each other. It was the talk of the hospital and I was not going to take responsibility for confirming a notice destined for the awesome *Times*.

The hospital was at the southern end of Goldhawk Road, close to Stamford Brook tube station, so there was easy access to the West End, but the river was even more beguiling. Apart from having to cross the Great West Road – busy but possible – the walk to the Thames was pleasant, through St Peter's Square and down Black Lion Lane, where the river itself, at all hours and tides, high or low, was special as only London River can be. I fear there was much missed which I would notice now but, as ever, I explored. Chiswick Mall, overlooking the river, was beautiful and away from the river I loved Chiswick House and tiny Chiswick Square.

Also in the area was The Dove, one of London's historic riverside pubs. Out with two friends one evening, I tried to jump over a railing; a 'crash barrier' in today's parlance, and hurt my knee. We still carried on with our walk, but the others suggested going into The Dove for a drink. The landlord was charming and even treated us to a free round. Even so I was acutely uncomfortable. Women did not go into pubs without male escorts. In fact I had once been taken to The Prospect of Whitby, the oldest and most famous of all London inns, but though pleased to see it, I could not relax despite having an escort, even despite being 'outside', on the old balcony with wonderful views of the Thames.

Our stretch of the river was part of the Boat Race course, but unfortunately not only was I on night duty, the tide meant the race was to be rowed at about 3 pm. That meant not enough sleep either before, or if I stayed up, after, and sleeping during the day was never easy. Two of us discussed going but decided not to and I slept well. Except that around 3 pm I woke up, thought 'Oxford's won' and went straight back to sleep. Double rejoicing, as normally it is impossible to get back to sleep once awake.

Half a dozen doctors were post-graduate students at Queen Charlotte's and quite often they joined us, adding fun to off-duty expeditions. At least twice a crowd of us went swimming in the river, out at Twickenham ferry. One of our set had trained at The London and she had a French boyfriend who owned an ice cream van. It was a long way for him to come out to Hammersmith, but one hot evening she persuaded him to arrive, quite late. Nine of us piled in, to sit rather uncomfortably on top of the fridges and worktops. Anne, an extrovert and inspirational character, did not have a swimsuit in London but she was undaunted. In bra, pants and a slip, topped by a wide brimmed straw sun hat, she was one to the first into the water. In no time, all we could see, in the moonlight, was a huge hat bobbing down the middle of the river, a vision treasured ever since.

More exams loomed, but one evening several unhappy doctors told us what had upset them in an exam they had taken that day. They were the post-graduates doing the obstetric course as academics, not housemen. We knew from our own studies that determining gender in some newborns could be difficult, but they had had a question on the subject with three hours in which to answer. What had upset them was the ambiguity of the wording, since it meant there were two ways to tackle the answer, but each one required three hours. Which did the examiners want? My reaction: there is that much complexity?!

This complaint made a great impression on me and I have quoted it more than once. Everyone has some male and female genes, but in a few cases the balance is wrong and in even fewer disastrously so. It is always heart rending to deliver a baby with any physical defect but must be peculiarly distressing to look at an apparently perfect new arrival and find indeterminate genitalia. Boy or girl? Worse, there may be internal problems with no external indications. The doctors' dilemma is a useful story, I think. Hopefully it arouses at least a little understanding for victims shunned by society.

Fortunately our own exams were much more straightforward. One written and one viva voce, but both in the fortnight following completion of our six months at Queen Charlotte's. We were offered the chance to work for that fortnight as staff nurses at Chelsea Hospital for Women, gynaecological branch of obstetric QCH. I jumped at the chance. After only five weeks doing midder I had decided to do Part II, but where? When at King's three people, independently, had all recommended that one should spend the total six months on the district, delivering babies in their own homes. Apart from the major cities, most schools only offered three months, the other three being spent in small hospitals or maternity homes, so my options were very limited.

By now I had had more than the longed for 'three-years-to-get-to-know-it' in London, and was anxious for some country life, preferably by the sea. Happily I was offered a vacancy in Plymouth, but not until December. Far from being a blow, I welcomed this, looking forward to spending the intervening month at home and planning to earn my living in some simple job completely different from nursing.

One morning I was on duty in Queen Charlotte's, the next in Chelsea, having moved lock stock and barrel from one nurses' home to the other, helped to speed on my way by friends not coming to Chelsea. I had acquired new uniforms and generally settled in. I was off duty from 11 am – 3 pm and went for quite a long walk, recording in my diary: 'This is a lovely area – very exciting.' The following day I met John. No longer was it just the area that seemed very exciting. From that day life itself took off into a stratosphere of excitement and joy.

Three Oxford graduates had collected their MAs – and telephoned our nurses' home hoping some nurses might join their celebrations. This ploy was not unknown and the friend who took the call yelled to me asking if I would like to go. Of course. The evening was voted very successful by all, not least the Albert Hall part.

At a Prom a couple of days earlier I had lost my purse and was getting ready to go and ask if it had been found when Joan called me. So the others all came too. We arrived in time to applaud Malcolm Sargent and shout encore with enthusiasm – but we had not heard a note. From there we went to John's flat in Pimlico, to listen to a Tom Lehrer record. He was an American Professor of Mathematics at Harvard, with a brilliant but iconoclastic and subversive wit, whose songs were banned by the BBC. He was wonderful.

So was John. We got on like a house on fire and agreed to go to the theatre together four evenings later. Two days later was my written exam and I went off to Queen's Square fortified by an amusing Good Luck card from John.

The building was enormous, an interesting place which seemed to be a dedicated examination centre. It was close to Bloomsbury and was part of the University of London. The atmosphere was not intimidating and I found it 'rather fun taking it with 777 other aspiring midwives'. One question I liked and for the only time in my life began the answer with a flippant remark. The question asked what would one expect to find if called to a railway station waiting room where a woman had just given precipitate birth, i.e. no warning – one contraction and there is the baby. I wrote that I would expect to find a very shocked mother and very shocked baby, but harder to diagnose what state the station staff would be in.

Ten days later our vivas were held in the same building. I was directed to one of a long row of small tables, where sat two examiners, a doctor and a midwife. They looked up with big smiles and to my horror they had in front of them my written paper! However, they were very kind and without actually saying so, left me in no doubt that I had passed.

That was supposed to be my last day in London. Nine days later I was back. By the end of our second meeting John and I were both wondering what had hit us. Incidentally, before we went to the theatre that evening he took me to Soho for my first ever Chinese meal. He made me eat all of it with chopsticks. I loved it. Chinese restaurants scarcely existed outside Soho – maybe one or two in Liverpool which had a small Chinese population – and even in Soho there were not many. Not quite so surprising then, that I had my first Chinese meal at the age of 23. That was on a Friday. Between then and the following Friday we met every day except one, and that evening he drove me home and stayed for the weekend. I had alerted (and frightened) my mother by asking for the handles on the sideboard to be changed. There is, obviously, a story behind this.

Before the war my parents had not finished furnishing their home and for several years afterwards only people who were newlyweds or had been bombed out were permitted to buy the limited utility furniture available. The trick was to buy second-hand and my mother was adept at identifying the most promising sources in the many small ads in the *Oxford Times*.

In 1947 many people were emigrating to Australia and we became friendly with the 'Paddys' – real surname Palmer, from whom we bought several things. They had a handsome sideboard which my parents coveted, though it was almost too big for our small house. It had been valued at £70, far too expensive for us. As sailing day approached the sideboard had still not been sold and the house clearance man had to be called in, notorious for taking advantage of such situations. My father told Paddy he could give him £10, in the unlikely event of less from the clearance firm. They offered £6 and the sideboard was ours. It was an indeterminate 1900/1920s design, made of heavy oak. Originally it had small drop metal handles on the cupboards and drawers. Someone had tried to modernise, with bright green thick plastic handles on the drawers, inappropriate and hideous.

It was intended that they should be replaced but, probably because there had been nothing available, the handles stayed put. Twelve years later they were no longer a screaming green anyway, having dulled with use to a less obtrusive greenish brown. Discussing them one day years before, I had joked that if bringing home THE man in my life, the only thing I would like changed in the house were those green handles. They were still in situ when Jenny and I sold the sideboard almost thirty years later.

Sideboard or no sideboard, I was blissfully happy and at the end of a week at home had abandoned the idea of working in Oxford. It was agreed I should go back to London, find a bedsit near John and find a job up there. On Sunday evening, 23 August, John drove me to Earl's Court to stay with friends. By Monday evening I had a job, had worked for half the day and had found a bedsit a couple of streets away from John's flat in Tachbrook Street, Pimlico.

In the morning I had gone to the Labour Exchange in Victoria and been sent to Thames Car Hire for what sounded like the ideal job. A receptionist to answer the phone and do a little typing. By lunch time I had been interviewed and accepted, met John and a friend for lunch and returned to the little office in John Adam Street, just off The Strand and beside Charing Cross Station. My employer promptly departed for home suffering from sciatica. Four visitors and one phone call did not fill the afternoon. Next day I became convinced that my hunch of the previous afternoon was right. He was unbusinesslike and in financial difficulties. By mid-week I felt pretty certain I would not be paid, nor was I. The invalid never appeared again and did not sound surprised when, at the end of the week in my daily phone call to report business, I told him I should not be returning next week. A trial week in more ways than one. Incidentally, to get to the office I had to go through a little bookshop. It, too, felt dodgy, with far too few customers to sustain it and an atmosphere as far from Blackwell's as could possibly be imagined. There were not even many books. The two men who ran it were pleasant to me in a perfectly ordinary way. Neither of them attempted to help me prise any money out of my hopeless employer but they did suggest going to an employment agency rather than the Labour Exchange as there were better jobs on offer. The Alfred Marks Employment Bureau near Victoria Station was one of a well-known chain at the time. The girls there were very nice and sent me to the Independent Order of Foresters in Cockspur Street, just off Trafalgar Square. Although with connections to archery, it was basically a sort of insurance, or Friendly Society. I started there at once, checking file cards to ensure that subscriptions had been entered correctly, a quarterly review duty, it was explained. The nine permanent staff did not have time, so temporary help was always employed. It was a happy office and I was made welcome. The work was not difficult but needed vigilance. It suited me, I rarely find detail too finicky or irritating. Unfortunately, the work was completed in a fortnight, together with another slightly different task. At the beginning of the third week I was promoted to using a typewriter, but when I finished a report the next day the manager, who had tried to find more for me to do, thanked me, shook my hand and said he had no more work. Tuesday lunchtime and no job. Off to Alfred Marks, but they had nothing. I rang John at his office – he was a Civil Engineer who designed things like dams and bridges – organised sandwiches and went off to queue for that evening's Prom. I was there so early we got seats by the fountain.

The Proms always remind me of how, when I was at school, my heart used to sink during their season. Day after day one opened the *Radio Times* to see the special box at the top of the page, profiling the programme for that evening. Not my taste. David had tried to educate me in some classical appreciation and at King's record evenings used to be organised for us. I only have two particular memories, the first of walking into the big, empty nurses sitting room at King's and hearing just a few minutes of Dvorak's *New World Symphony* on the radio. Could not wait to hear it all and have loved it ever since. The other time was when Peggy and I went to a concert one Sunday evening in the Albert Hall. We went to Evensong in St Mary Abbots Church in Kensington but slipped out before the sermon to rush up Kensington Gore for 7.30 pm. We heard Tchaikovsky's *1812 Overture*, complete with cannons, and ever since it has joined fun fairs as the only things which should be EXTREMELY NOISY – thinks she who loves silence. I still infinitely prefer live classical concerts rather than on TV, radio or records.

Alfred Marks could find no more temporary jobs for me. It was mid-September, holidays were over and, other than nursing, I had no skills to offer. The girls there were concerned on my behalf and by the end of the week were treating me to coffee and suggesting that they could easily teach me how to use a small manual telephone switchboard if necessary. They also decided that although I only had nine weeks left, the only solution was to send me to a permanent post. Hence, on the Friday, I went for an interview at Girl Guide Headquarters in Buckingham Palace Road. They needed a receptionist to sit in a small kiosk at the back entrance, monitoring visitors and receiving incoming goods. There was a stream of the latter, partly for the shop in HQ and partly for despatch to Guides all over the country. Having been accepted I started the following Monday, my third new job in five weeks.

There I stayed until it was time to leave for Plymouth. Boy Scouts HQ was next door, but they were treated as pariahs and regardless of them, I felt that if one wanted to find the Guiding spirit, Headquarters was not the place to look. In my lone cubby hole there were no problems and in the canteen for lunch I was welcomed to a table where a group of junior, though not very young, staff became good friends. They even gave me a memento when I left, a tiny tortoiseshell tortoise brooch.

Unfortunately, the overall pervading atmosphere to me seemed small-minded and narrow visioned, with far too many elderly spinsters around. Was I just being petty myself?

A rather unusual task given to me was designing the back pages of the weekly Guide, Guider, and Ranger magazines. It was a simple matter of arranging blocks, each featuring some piece of equipment for sale via HQ, but with sufficient flexibility to be interesting. I enjoyed that task, but not an associated incident.

All the staff, including the most senior, entered the building through the back door, passing my cubby hole. Apparently, one day I accosted Miss Norman with a query about the advertisements, as she arrived. She told me off, saying 'You wouldn't do that to your Matron, would you?' I was furious (it says in my diary). I bet I was. Writing this so many decades later later, the phrase that pops into my head is 'Silly old bat'; perhaps it should have been 'frustrated old spinster' – and I don't mean me. But she might have been one of many unfortunate women, akin to those who lost their chance of marriage due to the First World

War, now similarly afflicted by the Second. All the same, even now it is hard to believe that some folk take being told off in their stride.

It always upset me dreadfully, usually the slightest rebuke reducing me to jelly, but if I thought unjustified I burned with indignation. A telling-off never forgotten happened the previous year at the Baldwin Brown Convalescent Home near Camberley. Baldwin Brown was part of the King's group, staffed by permanent staff except for a couple of 'bonnets' who would be sent there for part of their fourth year. It should have been happy and relaxing, but was detested by every 'bonnet' who ever set foot in the place. In the spring I survived a fortnight there on relief duty, but in the summer had to return for an odd, badly organised mix of day and night duty. Meals in wards everywhere were rituals considered most important, being thought of as highlights in the patients' day. The wards were closed to visitors and doctors, patients sat up and made comfortable and the huge, heavy, heated food trolleys wheeled in. Sister took charge, carefully serving special diets sent from the diet kitchen or plating up helpings considered appropriate for each individual patient. Nurses waited with trays, ready to carry each meal to designated recipients. Trays were part of our lives. Tiny ones for medicines, slightly larger ones for drinks, bedside ones for water jug and glass, big ones for meals, huge ones for used crockery, stainless steel especially for dressings but in all sizes. Woe betide anyone caught not using a tray.

One lunch time at Baldwin Brown, Sister was in charge, but she asked me to serve the potatoes. They were quite small and the men were given three, until she told me to put two on the next plate for a man who needed a small helping. That done, I reverted to three for the next patient. She hit the roof. She had not told me to put three on that plate she ranted, though she knew as well as I did that the man in question had a healthy appetite.

At King's I had been told I was to be at Baldwin Brown for nine weeks. Counting the days, the ordeal was in the eighth week when Sister Kathleen, second in command, said something which made it clear she was expecting me for at least four more weeks after the nine were up. I sat down and wrote to Sister Joan at King's, explaining that I had tried to settle but found it impossible. She was the rather stern Deputy Matron whom Sister Kathleen suggested I write to. Is it possible Sister Kathleen was sympathetic? She was not as bad as the Sister in charge but that says little on her behalf. Next day there were hints from one of the nurses about my return to King's, 'various things had been said to make her think so'. She was right. There had been a phone call that afternoon and I was given my return date the following day. The prompt reaction was impressive indeed.

Back at King's my favourite admin Sister interviewed me. She asked quietly if I could explain why I had not liked it. I could not. Suddenly the potato episode and numerous other trivialities seemed far too petty to recount, so I stood silently in front of her feeling foolish. She gave me a kind, perceptive look and said, 'All right nurse, I know', and I left her office with a light heart.

One thing at Baldwin Brown which irked all the bonnets extremely was having to ask permission to give so much as an aspirin. This was not the arrogance of the newly qualified, nurses; on night duty we routinely made decisions about giving pain killers and sedatives.

During my senior night duty at the Wingfield it was my choice of barbiturates which were given at bedtime, often together with aspirin or codeine. Nowadays it is inconceivable that any nurse should have such responsibility, let alone an 18-year-old. Only DDAs, prescribed by doctors, had to be entered in the Dangerous Drugs Act register when administered, whether orally or by injection.

A final Baldwin Brown story before returning to Pimlico and John. On arriving there the first time, I was greeted at the door by a nurse who looked at the name on my suitcase and exclaimed, 'Are you a relative of the Brigadier?' Brigadier Sandilands lived next door!

I knew of his existence through seeing a letter he had written to the *Daily Telegraph*, but never imagined meeting him. One day I plucked up courage, gave my name to a puzzled butler who answered the door and was ushered in. The Brigadier was 80 years old, living with his 85-year-old Major General brother. They were classic retired army officers, quintessential bachelors both, courteous but unsure of how to cope with this unknown young woman. The second time at Baldwin Brown I actually lived in what had been their gardener's cottage. King's rented it from them for the night staff to live in – far from any cottage of my imagination, it was a spacious, pleasant, three-bedroom house of 1920 or '30s vintage, built at the road end of their long drive.

The Brigadier was delighted to think of me living there. We had a couple of pleasant encounters and he showed me big group photographs of his large family – umpteen nieces and nephews. He corresponded with my father, but at least as far back as 1812 they could find no family connection. However, their house was called Craibstone, the name of an estate near Aberdeen, which was familiar in our family tree. (As a direct result of a visit to explore Craibstone in 1991, I met my distant cousin, Pat Sandilands – and married him!! Guess the Brigadier would have been delighted.) Sadly the Major General was ill and deaf so I only met him once, briefly, but I treasure a photo with the two brothers which the Brigadier sent me.

Back to Pimlico. Petty or not, working at Girl Guide Headquarters was not a problem. Nothing was. John and I spent nearly every evening and all our weekends together. We went to concerts, theatres, cinemas, coffee bars, restaurants, spent many cheerful evenings with friends, including one in Trafalgar Square on election night, and at weekends drove to stay at my home, or his in Northamptonshire. His parents took us to a Rotary Club ball and John's sister and brother-in-law were good friends who lived in South Kensington. Life was full of love and fun.

Until a cloud at the beginning of November when, in a 'muddled way', John spoke of not being sure if he ever wanted to be married. Naturally, I was upset but mentally geared myself up for a long wait. Four weeks later, at home the night before I left for Plymouth, after much talking, it was all over. Well. Almost. Anguish followed, but during the first weeks in Plymouth I fought to keep in touch, writing many letters – to which John replied

Marriage would have been a disaster. John was the meanest man with money I have ever met. He disliked children. He particularly disliked the Church of England, of which I was a practising member. He preached tolerance but was intolerant of many things. While not a beer and sandals type of man, he detested formality, convention, tradition.

Brought up in a Quaker family, with a Quaker education, he had no Christian belief whatever but was an avowed pacifist. A firm for which he had hoped to work refused to insert a clause in his contract allowing him to opt out of any work which might, in any way, be connected with the armed forces or even defence. John had been very angry. I thought it their prerogative and stupid of him to try and dictate terms, especially as at the time he had been a young graduate seeking his first job. but I kept my opinion to myself. By the time we met he had seven years' experience, and salary, under his belt. This included working on a dam in some hot, very dangerous country, where the engineers lived in a guarded enclave. They earned enormous sums of danger money but had little on which to spend anything.

Despite all this, as usual it seemed fair to me to share expenses 50/50. With hindsight I realise he even exploited that at least once. The only time I ever saw him wear a suit was for an interview with his bank manager. His danger money was in an off-shore account but he was anxious to get it into England without paying tax on it. He said little afterwards but I had a notion that the manager had given him short shrift. By the time we parted my parents loathed him, but it was to be months before the scales dropped from my eyes. For many, many years I castigated myself for being so blind and immature. After all, I was 23 years old when all this happened, not a silly teenager. Then, in 2006, I went to a reception in the National Portrait Gallery in Edinburgh. It was a small party but full of interesting people, including a 'girl' who turned out to be past her fortieth birthday. We had a long chat about all sorts and somehow got on to the subject of boyfriends. I told her of my shame at my 23-year-old folly but she refuted it immediately, quoting several young colleagues at the V&A as well as herself at that age. Heartening to be so cheered and reassured.

Chapter 4

Plymouth
1959–1960

THERE IS MUCH to tell about my six months in Plymouth. Definitely a game of two halves. It began on a black, wet night which reflected my feelings exactly. To say it had been a difficult day is an understatement. After the trauma of the previous day I was in no state to face anyone, but in addition to meeting new folk in Plymouth, I was to break my journey in Bristol to join my grandparents and great aunt, for lunch at her house in Brislington. Leaving home to live so far away (220 miles – awful!) was bad enough; in Bristol I confided in my great-aunt but did not tell my grandparents. Perhaps I knew already that they too disliked John. We had spent a weekend with them and later they told my mother they were not happy – but still gave John a pound towards his petrol. We were on our way back to London when we saw a huge sign at Thruxton advertising pleasure flights. Five shillings and ten shillings. So into the airfield we turned, blew the petrol money and I revelled in my first ever flight. I know I did, though so excited cannot recollect a single detail. Was it a biplane? Did we sit beside or behind each other? Were we airborne for five or even ten minutes? No idea.

In the train from Bristol a youngish man talked to me for a long time. He had left his wife and family somewhere in the Midlands while he went to Plymouth hoping to start up a heating business, and have them join him later. Maybe he too was lonely and apprehensive, but I thought I sensed that he did it to be kind. Though not tearful – crying must be done in private – no doubt he could recognise an abject bundle of misery when he saw one. I never knew his name so could not look out for it but often hoped his fortunes thrived.

In Plymouth the pupil midwives shared a big house with District (Community) nurses in Durnford Street. Stonehouse was an historic area with some classic old buildings, including the Royal Marine Barracks directly opposite us. Some people had teased that I was going to Plymouth because of the Royal Navy, but when applying for Part II that thought never crossed my mind and after four months of loving a pacifist, any of the armed forces were the least of my concerns.

There were twelve pupils, six new ones every three months. Our rooms were small and dismal but we had a very pleasant sitting room where we spent most of our time. In those first weeks I made friends with Jenny in particular, although we all got on well with each other. Jenny confided an unhappy love affair recently ended and often I used to look at her and wonder which of us would disappear first, escaping to our room for a good cry.

One lucky girl had a car, one or two who also worked in the more distant suburbs travelled by bus, the rest of us cycled to our patients, not withstanding Plymouth's hills. My district, or rather Sister Cooper's district, was Lipson, quite near the city centre, so not too far, though my route lay along the notorious Union Street – every other establishment a pub – and up Royal Parade, the main post-war heart of the city. Plymouth had been blitzed to smithereens during the war and Devonport virtually obliterated, but much rebuilding had already been achieved by the time my set arrived. The city centre had been completely redesigned, with wide clean streets, very different from their forerunners. I was delighted to acquire two booklets with photographs of before, during and after, but was horrified by the scale of the destruction, despite knowing Bristol and London. There was an another route back to Stonehouse, away from Royal Parade, round by the sea at the foot of Plymouth Hoe, which as an alternative was a great pleasure.

Lipson was mainly an area of little streets lined with small terraced houses, but it also included a park at the top of which was a terrace of huge houses, considered the best address in the city. One of my first deliveries was in one of these houses. A third baby arrived three weeks early – and four days before the mother's friend was available to undertake her promise to look after her. It meant the father had to cope with wife, new baby and the two older children. He was incensed. I never met a more resentful man, who made it clear the work was beneath his dignity. Poor wife. The idea that father should be present at the birth was in its radical infancy. With no concessions whatever I was keen to have all fathers watch the arrival of their offspring, but my splendid Sister Cooper, while not totally opposed, certainly did not encourage it. In my six months I delivered more babies (thirty-six) than anyone else in my set, with only having to transfer two or three mums to hospital. Sister would sit on the bed doing her knitting, rub backs during contractions and cheerfully encourage. She was well known and liked in the area, trusted and down to earth, so the mums relaxed and all was well.

At first, for many weeks the rain was relentless. On Christmas morning I had three post-natal visits and stood on the first doorstep sodden and dripping, wetter than ever, but as always and everywhere, was welcomed – except by the unhappy man at the posh address.

In the New Year Jenny received a hamper of food from her father and a letter telling her to have a party with some of her men friends. That puzzled her twice over; first, because it was so out of character for her father to suggest such a thing, and second – she did not know any men in Plymouth anyway. Sue did.

A fellow pupil, her home was in Yelverton, in other words she was a local girl and would organise some men from Manadon. The name meant nothing and Jenny was in no mood to care, but the party was organised and the men turned up. How Sue had come to know them became a legendary tale.

She and her sister went up to London for a day's shopping, travelling overnight on the train, returning the following evening, arriving back in the early hours. On the way up a couple of guys pestered them, so when, during the return journey, two more tried to be friendly, the girls were very shirty. Being Naval officers, however, these two persisted and by the time the train reached Plymouth Sue and Anthea had agreed to go to a tiddly-winks match with them. From that inauspicious beginning I lost count after seven weddings and twenty-one babies. The boys were at HMS *Thunderer*, the Royal Naval Engineering College at Manadon in the north of the city. They were part of Fifty Eight Long Course, a group of twenty-two officers on a three-year degree course. At some point one of their instructors told us they were considered an exceptionally bright bunch, which was surely true. At least two of them became Admirals and nearly all of them were talented – certainly at planning innumerable ways of having fun.

Just before Jenny's party, when we first met some of them, Jenny read her father's letter again and realised he had written 'have a party with some of your *new* friends'. Too late...

I was one of her bridesmaids when she became one of those seven brides the following year. By then I had fallen in love with the entire Royal Navy and my heart still lifts when I see one of His Majesty's ships out in the bay beyond my home.

First I had many more hours of misery over John to endure, losing one-and-a-half stone in the process.

And I have not yet mentioned Devil's Point...

Nowadays Devil's Point is a public park with paths, benches and information boards; in 1960 it was a seldom visited headland of deserted gun emplacements and tangled undergrowth.

The name is doubtless due to the vicious rocks edging the sea all around. Happily, there are stunning views across Plymouth Sound to Staddon Heights, Drake's Island and Mount Edgecumbe from the land above them, but, most exciting, close-ups of the currents where the River Tamar enters the Sound. Local boatmen warned that seven different currents meet there. After the balloon of river above Cremyll, vast amounts of water have to squeeze through the narrow gap between Mount Edgecumbe and the Point. The patterns of strong tidal currents are mesmerising, with a sense of concealed energy adding to their power of inexplicable attraction. Small boats have to choose the state of the tides with care.

It was almost disappointing to watch Ark Royal come in one day, scything her way through the high water with apparent disdain. I went down there innumerable times, morning, noon and night. On my way back from deliveries, after parties, feeling unutterably miserable, feeling elated; on foot, on bicycle or in friends' cars. It was my place. When I went to see it again in 1999 what a shock it was to discover how many holidaying hordes it had to be shared with, but they – together with the new manicured tidiness – did not spoil it. The magic was still there, originally found as a surprise at the far end of Durnford Street when first exploring as a newly arrived pupil.

We pupils lived much nearer the end that joined Union Street, in a huge, ugly hostel but looked after by a marvellous married couple. Our meals were superb, far better than any other nurses' homes I ever stayed in, so it was doubly sad that my constant requests were for small helpings or none at all. Baked Alaska was one of Mrs Harris' specialities – ultra fashionable at the time but astonishing in a nurses' home – yet even that rarely tempted me. The pupils all sat together at one long table, with our tutor at the head serving the food. Not exactly a mild form of torture, but difficult. Until after lunch one Thursday.

By then, despite John's words before I left home, foolishly I had harboured a hope that our relationship might be rekindled. For one exhausting day I had gone up to London on the overnight train to see him on his birthday, and then we met on my one long weekend off, which I had chosen to have exactly halfway through my six months, at the end of February. It was during that visit John told me plainly that he would not marry me, ever.

So the second half of Part II started in wretchedness – a carbon copy of three months earlier. Except that the relentless rain had stopped. We were at the beginning of one of the most beautiful three months of the twentieth century, a never to be forgotten spring in that unrivalled part of the world for spring, Devon.

Two months after the first party with boys from HMS *Thunderer*, we had a second one. Six days after that, in mid-March, Jenny and I saw a boat for sale – and less than five weeks after that I wrote in my diary that I felt as if I were just delivering babies in my spare time.

District midwifery, for several decades, involved much time 'on call', i.e. when on duty, being at home within hearing of the telephone. No mobile phones or radio call systems in 1960. Patients had alternative numbers to ring if their own 'booked' midwife was not available. It was being 'on call' which allowed us time for the boat, about which more later.

First, a bit more about domiciliary midwifery.

Historically the development of midwifery as a profession was very different from nursing, and for many years officialese referred to 'Nursing and Midwifery'. Apart from any other details, qualified midwives, unlike nurses, are practitioners in their own right, though it was illegal for patients not to be registered with a doctor also. Attendance at a residential, week long refresher course every five years was mandatory, and the guidelines of the Midwives Code of Practice clear. Formal registration of midwives began in 1902. The registration of nurses only followed some twenty years later, as Florence Nightingale had been opposed to it.

As this is not a treatise on midwifery I have no intention of detailing the stages of labour or possible difficulties. However, it is fact that complications such as haemorrhage, though very rare, can occur with dramatic speed and danger. Hence the wisdom of 100 per cent deliveries in hospital as recommended by Sir John Peel in his 1960 Report. Sir John was a KCH Consultant and the Queen's obstetrician after the sad, sudden death of the much loved Sir William Gilliatt, with whom Sister Rowe had worked.

Pregnant mothers chose where they wanted to be delivered, and the less educated chose overwhelmingly to stay at home, due to fear of hospitals. It was considered wise for first babies to be delivered in hospital as they are a bit of an unknown quantity, but it was certainly not essential. Long before 1960, breech deliveries at home were rare and unwise, but when one baby obviously intended to arrive feet first, a GP with confidence in my midwife, Sister Cooper, told her to carry on. Having been a breech myself (my mother in hospital) I was delighted, though apprehensive, at this unexpected chance, but with Sister supervising did it by myself. Happily, it was a small baby and all was well. Normally, even in hospital the doctors did the breech deliveries, so for me an extremely rare, fortunate opportunity. After deliveries we did post-natal visits morning and evening for three days, then mornings only for the next seven. Diary entry: 'Big fuss by Sister yesterday when she found Mrs Watson up for two hours on her fourth day.' (!!!)

I cannot remember any problems which ever needed more frequent visits, not even feeding. Physiologically breastfeeding is part of having a baby, and the uterus, for example, demonstrably reverts to normal size more quickly, but bottle feeding was all too often thought easier.

After ten days Health Visitors were responsible for the supervision of baby care. They ran baby clinics throughout the city and as part of our training we went to several 'Infant Welfare Clinics'. An exasperated entry in my diary complains about the heartbreaking job of trying to teach dim-witted mums how to look after their babies.

We had no liaison of any sort with the local maternity units, and our lectures were all at Durnford Street.

Each pupil worked with one midwife who covered a designated district. Everyone had one day off a week, and on Sister's day off her pupil would report to her deputy. Often just one formal phone call, as we usually did post-natal visits on our own.

Often on my own day off, in pre-boat weeks, I would go for long cycle rides. One afternoon I returned from a long expedition on Dartmoor to hear that Prince Andrew had arrived. Delivered by Sir John Peel and cared for by Sister Annette, also from King's.

Babies notoriously favouring the night hours to begin their arrival, we had a duty room with telephone for taking night time calls. We had a rota for sleeping in there, one night at a time. If the call was for the person on duty, she called a friend to take over her bed. One night three different people slept in the same sheets. An older pupil, a lovely woman in her forties, whose RAF fiancé was killed in the war, was incensed by the system. She succeeded in getting it stopped, so when in the duty room we were not to be called out. In practice the phone seldom rang, but peaceful night or not, none of use ever slept through the Royal Marines 6 am Reveille bugle in the Stonehouse Barracks directly opposite us. We spent some happy times with them in their theatre – a proper one, quite large, with the RM badge on the drop curtain, and some hilarious productions when it was raised.

It was an afternoon in mid-March that Jenny and I first saw the boat. The two of us had walked down the street to Cremyll Bridge to see the Duke of Edinburgh who was on a visit to Plymouth. He was to drive to Devonport to leave on a helicopter, but the cloud was low, the flight cancelled, and the Duke never appeared. By chance, I happened to look down from the bridge to the head of Stonehouse Creek, where there was a sign beside one of the boats. FOR SALE £12. It was badly in need of a coat of paint, but something made me go down and talk to the owner of the boatyard, Mr Adams, who said I could have her for £10, and a free berth.

After doing evening visits I went to see Mr Easton, the boat owner, who told me that the craft had no oars or rowlocks – so we shouldn't buy it! I had hoped Jenny would agree the purchase but she was away for her long weekend. A few days later I went back to the boatyard to thank Mr Adams for his help and Jenny came with me. He told us he would fix oars and rowlocks for us and suggested seeing Mr Easton again, asking if he would accept £9.

Two days later Jenny and I were the delighted owners of a twelve foot, wooden clinker-built, rowing boat of unknown age. Presumably at some point someone had mentioned seaworthiness?

From then on life changed quite dramatically, our days endlessly busy and full of fun. We could work on the boat when on call because we were near enough to be fetched quickly if needed, and the rain which plagued our first three months gave way to three months of glorious weather. We had no end of help from all our friends, and we scraped off old paint, stuffed putty in holes and brushed on new paint. We would arrive to do more work and find somebody else had already done something extra. The local boatmen helped, the boys from Manadon helped, and everyone was interested. Except one pernickety midwife, noted for being difficult, who unlike all the others forbade her pupil to go to the boat, insisting it was too far from the telephone.

We needed a name for it. Everyone liked 'Hydramnios', but we decided it might suggest water inside the boat, which was not a good idea. We were sure we wanted a midwifery term of some sort but a suitable one was elusive. Eventually we settled on HEROS ½ – i.e. Her os (cervix) half dilated; that is, making good progress in labour. How we ever thought that one up, let alone chose it, is a mystery, but we liked it – and it provoked our tutor, nicknamed 'Aunty', to make her only joke in six months. Aunty was a small, round, earnest middle-aged spinster who was not a gifted teacher. Our amazement cannot be overstated when she asked about the name and commented, 'After all your hard work I am surprised it is only half dilated'!

The name was beautifully painted for us by someone at Manadon, and we began to plan a launching party. Jenny's midwife was the friend and colleague of my midwife,, so we were pleased when they agreed to perform the ceremony. Sister Dodd would smash a bottle of Babycham over the bow, and Sister Cooper would declaim: 'I name this boat Heros ½ and may all who row in her be able to swim.'

Incidentally, in the first letter from my mother after writing to her about this enterprise, she ended a few dubious comments with: 'If you do buy it, always keep one foot on dry land.'

For the party we decided on a barbecue, and were heading towards inviting the world and his wife. In those days the grassy, rather derelict far side of the creek had plenty of space so was ideal. Today it is lined with glossy waterfront flats. Such a pity.

Only an hour or so before the party Jenny suffered her 'humper bite'.

Sue had just passed her driving test and was reversing her new pride and joy with Jenny watching her. No reflection on Sue's driving; Jenny just stood there too long and the bumper hit her on the shin. Someone later trying to explain the accident said 'the humper bit her', and the spoonerism it was ever after. The 'bite' was actually a very large lump which took twelve months to absorb and disappear, meantime Jenny came to the BBQ feeling battered and fragile.

In the previous weeks we had heard from the Manadon boys much concern for Archie, an Australian in their group who was in hospital for several weeks with kidney problems. He was discharged on the day of the BBQ, and the two invalids sat quietly together for most of the evening.

I was a bridesmaid at their wedding twelve months later.

The party went well, though our intended row after the launch began ignominiously. Jenny was able to climb in despite her leg injury – but we both managed to face the wrong way… A greetings telegram from home read 'Happy times. Warn lifeboat to stand by.'

We had sent an invitation to the editor of the *Western Evening Herald*, who sent a reporter and gave us a long write-up, and photograph, in the paper. We hoped it would amuse our patients, though did any of them notice that the name of the boat was not reported?

Though it was in the photograph. Anyway, it was kind to give us so much space. We had told the reporter of our gratitude for all the help we were given, but did not mention things like arriving one day to find the boat turned upside down, with two large tins of paint underneath. In the next six weeks or so, until the end of our training, we had a lot of fun rowing around in the creek, and also two real expeditions. One day we rowed across to Cremyll and enjoyed a walk on the Cornish side of the Tamar, on another, four of us went out to Drake's Island in the Sound. I cannot remember any concern about the tidal currents at Devil's Point, but as two Naval officers were with us no doubt we felt safe, though we did worry a bit when a Customs launch seemed to be chasing us. Rumour had it that the island was closed to the public, but no one really knew. We landed on the side away from the main channel, and spent a happy afternoon clambering around, and in, the massive old fortifications. Jenny had organised a picnic, including strawberries and Cornish cream – calorific intake useful as the tide had gone out and we had to haul the boat several feet down to the water. She was heavy, and the drag was quite a challenge. A big shock was seeing all the exposed rocks, which we had just missed when arriving…

At some point we learnt that Archie was not Archibald, but Anthony. His nickname was short for 'Arch Bastard', acquired at the Australian equivalent of Dartmouth due to his efforts to make his colleagues get up when it was his turn to wake them. Dartmoor, and Devon pubs both moorland and coastal, gave us many happy hours. On one cheerful day we picnicked and played Pooh Sticks after climbing Vixen Tor. The Australians had never heard of Pooh Sticks and they loved it. To get to Vixen Tor we had had quite a long trek over open, tussocky moorland. An abiding memory is one of the boys having an enormous coil of climbing rope slung round him from one shoulder, but with not a boulder, let alone a rock face, in sight. Eventually Vixen Tor appeared and then my first, and last, attempt at rock climbing. I got so well stuck in a simple, thirty foot chimney that serious thought began as to how I could be rescued from this narrow gully. It was shame which forced me to extricate myself somehow, and I reached the top. Have no idea how I got down.

Another happy expedition was an excellent car rally out on Dartmoor, chasing the Green Man along small lanes. Given a list of clues, most were located and solved but one remained largely a mystery. On a small table in the middle of nowhere – itself needing to be found – a drink was set up to be identified. People who tried it were not impressed, and only one person was successful. Cornish Mead. Not a good advertisement for it, despite being part of a lot of fun.

Meals out were always a treat. and a small mistake in a waterside pub in Kingsbridge – hugely helpful and never forgotten. In a large party several of us chose steak, and as ever I played safe and ordered medium. They arrived with small flags delineating rare, well done, etc. Mine turned up flagged very rare. In such a crowd nothing to be done. No one was calling for a lost very rare; complaining, or sending back, was unthinkable.

The very rare steak proved to have infinitely more flavour than any cooked for longer. After almost sixty years a very rare fillet steak remains the treat at the top of my list of favourite food, preferably with Béarnaise sauce. (Essential the beef is top quality.)

(NB. In 1966 the well trained waiters on the SS *Oriana* told me the correct term was 'blue', but seldom recognised. Too true. Until recently, decades later, when asking for my very rare annual treat, it is now likely to be queried, or corrected, 'Blue?' Yes, please!)

Above all, the fun in our sun-filled spring was the thrill of sailing for the first time. Six of us went out in 'Sir Galahad', a 30ft yacht belonging to the College.

We were not supposed to go beyond the breakwater, but the man on duty agreed not to report us and we set off for the Eddystone. It was perfect weather, but the lighthouse reef is seventeen miles out and the boys eventually decided to turn back. To my surprise I was allowed to helm, and left at the tiller from the breakwater right round past the Hoe, Drake's Island and Devil's Point, into the Tamar. Suddenly Ted appeared and exclaimed 'We're going to hit that buoy!' It was some way off beam so with confidence this greenhorn said 'No, we're not.' 'Yes, we bloody well are,' said the sailor, flinging the tiller out of my hand. The strong tidal stream would have driven us straight on to it – and right below the Admiral's house.

Ever since, I have thought Ted's apology for swearing was uncalled for. If ever swearing was justified…

Six months in Plymouth completed our midwifery training, with only the Part II exam to follow. We finished in May, but 1960 continued to be an eventful year.

First Jenny and I had a week's holiday in Falmouth, thanks to Jenny's parents who drove down from Tipton in the West Midlands to take us. The family had often holidayed there, and for six months Jenny had been a staff nurse in the local hospital before coming to Plymouth, so she knew the area well and took me exploring. At the end of a happy week we caught 'The Cornishman' express from Truro to Bristol, enjoying a delicious lunch in the dining car after standing at the windows when going through Plymouth, to look at 'our' districts.

We stayed overnight with my grandparents in Midsomer Norton before next day taking ourselves to Southmead Hospital (outskirts of Bristol) for our Part II exam – a practical.

First we each had a pregnant patient to examine. Mine was a woman who was an in-patient during her second pregnancy, but any examination always begins with taking a history. There was a lot to talk about as she had had a difficult time with her first baby. She was very pleasant and all went well. We had finished before the bell went, and then she said she was just wondering if there was anything else she could tell me. 'Oh, I know. I am in now due to having high blood pressure.' As in our Part 1 exams we sat at a table facing a midwifery tutor and a male Consultant. When I arrived for my inquisition the first question was, 'Why was my patient in hospital during this pregnancy?' In one answer I mentioned posterior positions – notably tricky. The midwife gave me a hard time quizzing about them. The Obstetrician, who was far easier, was inclined to make a statement and all I had to do was agree. Tutor not happy. At the end he said 'Very nice'. so I departed with my fingers crossed.

Shortly after this relatively straightforward ordeal I was in the grip of a nightmare which became a horrible panic. Jenny's exam was running late and I was tasked with phoning Manadon to give a warning message, as Tony was to meet her train. Bristol was the first city to have the new STD phone system, inaugurated by the Queen not long before, and like most non-Bristolians I had never used it. The system got the better of me, and I lost my only sixpenny coin. Not often do I panic, but trying to acquire another sixpence then use it successfully, was an episode not to be repeated. Fortunately it was second time lucky. And Jenny caught the train anyway.

A few days later my SCM Certificate arrived. Seven years after starting my training I was a qualified nurse and midwife, entitled to put nine letters after my name.

SRN (State Registered Nurse) **SCM** (State Certified Midwife) **ONC** (Orthopaedic Nursing Certificate) – only given on completion of SRN training.

Chapter 5

National Cash Register Co. London
1960–1961

WITHIN A FORTNIGHT of the start of my Part II training, I had agreed to return to London to share a flat with Jenny, who had never been there. A few weeks later it was Jenny who found a job for me. With many ideas about what not to do, I had only vague positive ones, of which industrial nursing was one.

Jenny had spotted an advertisement for a nurse at the head office of the National Cash Register Co. (NCR), which I applied for, was given an interview and was accepted. Future settled.

On 1 July 1960 I started my job as an industrial nurse in the Medical Department at the UK head office, in Baker Street (main HQ Dayton, Ohio, USA). Sister Gate was my boss; a middle-aged spinster but not at all spinsterish and very nice.

We were the only two nurses at HQ. When introduced to the Personnel Manager on my first day, rightly or wrongly, it seemed the time to ask if I could have a half day on 29 July, as I have been invited to a Naval Ball in Plymouth. I felt awful, being so new, but had to ask at some point, and the invitation had to be answered. They were very kind, and all was well.

By now two significant things had happened since leaving Plymouth. Aunt Sheila – the kind but formidable sister of my father – had turned up, and Jenny and I were sharing a flat in Pimlico.

How we came to share the flat with Pat Irvine, whom we had never met, I cannot remember. Jenny was clever, and was to do high-powered chest nursing at the Brompton hospital, a major chest diseases centre – and Pat midwifery at the Westminster. Pat had a sister, Liz, already living in London. Aunt Sheila, via a few problems, found the flat for us, but when she drove me to 13 Cambridge Street, I protested and said that this is where Liz lives.

By a phenomenal coincidence we three were in the basement, Liz and five others on the top two floors and two more nurses on the ground floor.

We soon became a London base for some of the Manadon boys, and I tried hard, but unsuccessfully, to fall in love with Warwick. He and Archie – now Tony – came down to Falmouth one day during our week there, and later Jenny told me it had been Warwick's idea. Next, when at home before going to London, he wrote a long letter to me, then phoned and asked to come and see me. Aunt Sheila was with us when he rang. Very disapproving of an Australian until I happened to say something about when he was at Dartmouth. 'Oh, was he at Dartmouth?', and instantly he was acceptable. I forbore to tell her that by 1958 all Naval Officers went to Dartmouth.

When I went down to the Summer Ball it was a shock when Warwick told me he was falling in love with me, having been certain he was someone who would just be a friend.

After suddenly switching off distress about John months before, I rang him soon after settling in Cambridge Street. He was to return my twenty-first birthday present table lamp and a few other things, lent to him for his new flat in the basement of his sister's house. He came for a meal, did not impress Jenny or Pat, and I wondered what on earth I had ever seen in him.

Warwick's father, Commander Raymont, was in London; also in the RAN, he was Australian Naval Attaché to the UK. In the autumn he was a patient in Chatham Naval hospital and one day Warwick drove me down to visit him, via an hour-long and five-mile traffic queue to cross the Medway bridge. No bypass or motorway then. Commander Raymont fussed repeatedly about getting a cup of tea for us, clearly having a problem. Not many weeks later he died with a brain tumour.

Warwick was an only child, his parents divorced and he had no contact with his mother. Even before his father's death his drinking worried me. I never saw him under the influence of alcohol, and wonder if I overreacted. He was tall. charming, fun, and someone said he was the most eligible bachelor of 300 men at Manadon.

The following year in Torquay I enjoyed his wedding to my flatmate Pat.

Also that autumn Jenny and Tony got engaged. Missing the Trafalgar Day Dinner in College was a henious crime, but Tony had skipped it to see Jenny. His excuse to his Commander was that he was proposing to his girlfriend.

We were in the Cambridge St. flat for nine months, with lots of socialising, including with the girls in the rest of the house. In our basement we had an excellent Hallowe'en party with various decorations including black cut-out footprints stuck across the ceiling. My boss, Sister Gate, enjoyed herself but arrived very late. She had a lift with two young men and they got lost, but had so much fun she was already in party mood, although they had not stopped at any pubs to ask the way.

One day Pat and Jenny gave me a talking-to. I must stop wearing pyjamas and start wearing nighties. More feminine. I disliked the idea, having always worn pyjamas (never called PJs) but did as I was told, and have never worn pyjamas since.

One evening in the flat upstairs, I watched with astonishment as Pat and Liz made a curry. We were getting ready for a party and the two sisters were each going round and round the big kitchen table. With no scales or other measuring kit, one would say to the other 'I've put sultanas in'; or nuts, or nutmeg, or baked beans, or left-over vegetables…

They just went on and on and it sounded awful. I dreaded supper. It was delicious. Great lesson and useful ever since.

At NCR I went out to our factories at Brent and Elstree as cover when their own nurse was on holiday. Safety care was good and there was little to do.

At Head office I enjoyed the secretarial side, with much filing of medical certificates and other paperwork, but as far as nursing was concerned even giving an injection was a major event. Frequent medical examinations of new employees were pretty dull and routine and I began to get restless. Pat used to come home full of tales, hilarious and otherwise, from her midder at the Westminster, sparking memories of enjoying mine.

Passing written exams was relatively easy but I was always slow at practical work. Although aware of not being the nurse I would like to be, I felt that even I was capable of more than the work at NCR.

Ward sisters had always terrified me, and I never, ever, wanted to be one. Nor was being one enjoyable, but that fate lay twenty years in the future.

Midwifery, on the whole, was different, as internal rotation often meant that no ward was the single fiefdom of one Sister. Anyway, when Pat announced that she intended to return to Devon (her home was in Torquay), to work in the Maternity Unit at Freedom Fields Hospital in Plymouth, it was an easy decision to join her.

Jenny and Tony were getting married at Easter, so we would all leave the flat together. Jenny asked me to be her bridesmaid, and my dress was made in Bond Street!

Her father footed the bill. The measuring was complex but one visit amused me, and made the others laugh when I told them: 'Point a Point' was nipple to nipple.

Chapter 6

Freedom Fields Hospital Maternity Unit Plymouth

1961–1965

FOUR YEARS IN Plymouth were not particularly exciting in retrospect, though I loved the city, the surrounding country and the sea, imagining myself staying there indefinitely.

Pat was only at Freedom Fields for eight weeks before leaving to get married, which did not endear her to the Superintendent Midwife. As soon as her intention was known she was put on night duty, which did not endear the Superintendent Midwife to her. It seemed reasonable to me but of course I never said so.

Jenny and Tony were living in a married quarter out at Crownhill, nearer Dartmoor. They gave me a lift to Torquay for the wedding, a big one, but nothing special remembered about it, except that Pat had a lovely dress and made a beautiful bride. What I do remember is being back in my room in the Nurses' Home by 6 pm. It was a bleak evening.

After a dull year living in the Nurses' Home, a friend, Maureen Young, agreed to share a flat with me. We found an ideal one, within easy walking distance of the hospital. It was on the first floor of a tall Victorian terraced house in Connaught Avenue, Mutley Plain, a useful suburban shopping area. We loved it.

Freedom Fields had two Obstetric consultants, and their standard was excellent. Only two storeys high and quite modern, the Maternity Unit had a lying-in ward on each floor, one for each consultant, though not totally exclusive in busy times. The wards were divided into rooms with four beds and curtains on rails, unlike the wooden ones at the Wingfield in my early training days. The big nurseries were opposite, on the other side of the corridor, all babies were put in them at night. Post-natal mums stayed for ten days. Ostensibly to establish breastfeeding, and to rest and recover from delivery.

When the dictate arrived that all babies must stay beside their mothers at all times, the midwives protested vehemently. New mothers needed sleep. Remote scientists, concerned by bugs seen through microscopes, impractical and clueless about real life, were concerned about cross-infection. We never had any such problems since a good level of general cleanliness was maintained.

The ten days gave way for two reasons. The mothers often hated it, being away from home for so long, and a few even took their own discharge. The other reason was the explosion in the birth rate already mentioned. It put huge pressure on units elsewhere, and so forty-eight hour discharge was invented in Bradford – it did not take long to become normal all over the country.

An asset was having our own operating theatre, so emergency caesareans were never delayed by general theatres all being in use. All the midwives would scrub as necessary, one to assist the surgeon and one to take the baby. To my surprise I enjoyed both, but especially assisting the surgeon. Taking the baby could be stressful if sir or madam refused to breathe, but it was rare indeed to have that problem for more than seconds or a minute, though that could feel an age, and one held one's own breath until the welcome first gasp – or indignant holler.

Staffing pressures were seldom, but when on duty in the delivery rooms babies deciding to arrive ten in one night or none in another, made life unpredictable. It was this that yet again provoked theorists into action, with the invention of planned delivery dates via labour induction. Deliveries would take place during daytime hours, Monday to Friday, when all the ancillary staff were on duty; obstetricians, paediatricians, radiographers, cleaners etc.

A friend of my sister went to booking clinic in Oxford and was astonished to be given the date the baby was to be born. Instinctively I felt there was a flaw in this and of course there was. Despite inductions babies often persisted in arriving 'out of hours'.

Much worse was that induction caused more painful labour, as mothers witnessed if having had previous normal labours. Longer, too,

71

as nature was not ready for the baby to be born. I was lucky to avoid this distressing nonsense, thanks to working with obstetricians who did not endorse unnecessary inductions. When a practising midwife I do not remember hearing the medical phrase 'Meddlesome Midwifery', but as a mantra for avoiding bad practice it is cheering wisdom.

Incidentally, the possibility of litigation never crossed our minds. This nasty, damaging idea that a poor experience must automatically be the fault of someone, who must be made to pay up large sums of money, has crossed the Atlantic as one of America's most destructive, and expensive, practices. How on earth a lawyer has the expertise to understand the huge variables of childbirth is a mystery to me.

Gross negligence in my day was so negligible as to be virtually non-existent, and nowadays is not the cause of the wholesale fear of legislation. Simple misunderstandings by unhappy parents fuel the rush to law, hence the forms bureaucracy invented in case evidence is required, an unforgivable major time-filling exercise.

After I had been at Freedom Fields for two years our Maternity Matron sent for me one day and to my astonishment said it was time I was a Sister!

She wanted me to go to Devonport Maternity Home, one of two ancillary units in the city. To get to Devonport, on the other side of the city from Mutley Plain, meant two bus journeys which took a minimum forty minutes, and people began to say I needed a car.

When first back in Plymouth learning to drive had seemed a sensible thing to do, purely because I thought it might be useful in an emergency – in someone else's car. It certainly never occurred to me that I might own a car of my own.

At the time several girls were learning to drive, taught by Mr Kendall, an ex-Metropolitan Police Flying Squad driver – better known as The Sweeney. However after twenty-two lessons I gave up, having taken the driving test twice and failed more badly the second time.

Eighteen months later, in the space of two hours one morning, I became the owner of a brand new Mini, a bank loan and a provisional driving licence.

My father and others had insisted I buy the best second-hand car I could afford and it must be from a reputable dealer. Several Manadon boys had mentioned a garage they used. It turned out to be in a back street not far from Connaught Avenue, and when our landlord told me to go there – and rang them – no more recommendation was needed. Off I went, and the first question was 'How much can you afford?' £120 was the honest answer, but it seemed far too little and I told the biggest fib ever and said £400. No idea where that was to come from! But Mrs Robins, the proprietor, astonished me. She took me to the little showroom, waved her hand towards a brand new Mini, saying it was £530 but she could let me have it for £500.

No doubt she recognised me for a green-un, and asked if I was in good standing with my bank. I replied that I thought so, and was soon there asking for a loan. Granted, by the deputy manager. A fortnight later the manager returned from holiday and sent for me. Most unpleasant and displeased, he declared he would not have given me the loan, and read the riot act about not keeping up payments, implying that nurses were unreliable.

I was angry and should have told him in no uncertain terms that I would never have asked for a loan if unable to keep up the payments. But I did not, never having been much good at standing up for myself.

Perhaps I should have remembered NCR. When I arrived to work there, Sister, and the company doctor, told me – 'so that I could stick my chest out' – that I had been chosen out of ninety-six applicants. Deflation of my chest followed when preparing to leave however.

This time there were 106 replies to the *Nursing Times* advert, but most were so dreadful it was hard to pick out a shortlist of six. Some applications were written on paper torn out of notebooks, some with appalling handwriting, almost all with bad grammar and some virtually illiterate. More than one explained why it was important for them to be given the job, citing various personal circumstances. What an eye-opener. It was hard to believe they were qualified nurses. Would all of them have been financially reliable? Probably an unworthy thought, but perhaps the bank manager had experienced a reason for his diatribe.

The car was an Austin Mini, YDR 521. Pretty pale grey/blue colour. A week after the 'Day of the Car' I had a week's holiday. My father came down by train, collected the car while I was on duty, and next day we set off for Oxford, with my sister in the back. She had been staying with me for a couple of days after a holiday job sailing.

The A38 in Devon in those days was an awful road, narrow, hilly and with numerous bends.

Part way to Exeter Daddy pulled into a lay-by, said it was my car and I must drive, so no option. Jenny said she was feeling ill by the time we got home...

My father took me out every day, then returned with me to Plymouth.

Next, back to Mr Kendall. At the end of the lesson he announced 'Well, Miss Sandilands, now you drive as if you belong behind the wheel, instead of being surprised to find yourself there!' He was absolutely right. Interesting that I found the Mini far easier than his quite big dual-control Rover, which he had always contended was easier to learn in, being a larger, smoother car.

After only four more lessons I took the test again. When wanting an emergency stop the examiner would bang the dashboard. He did. I stopped – and nearly put him through the windscreen (just a short time before seat belts.) He was impressed, and at the end he was very kind, telling me 'some people pass as they are just competent, but with me he felt very relaxed and enjoyed a drive round the town. He had total confidence in me.' Wow!

I have enjoyed driving ever since, not least in Europe, the US and New Zealand. When Mr Kendall got back in the car after the test his first remark was that the next step was to take my Advanced test. Not quite the next, but twenty-two years later I took it in Cyprus, where a thriving branch of the Institute of Advanced Motorists (IAM) helped many of us. Examiners used to fly out from the UK, and the man who examined me knew Mr Kendall. The IAM had many ex-police in the organisation – men keen on road safety. Apparently to many people any word of police involvement is an automatic turn off; such a shame.

(Talking of driving and of Cyprus, it was there that I won two driving competitions in one weekend, but more of that later.)

For now, back to Plymouth. Or, more accurately, away from Plymouth – first on a sailing holiday, second on a camping holiday, third on departing for pastures new.

Sailing Holiday

After several months at Freedom Fields a letter arrived out of the blue from Ted – he of the justified swearing. He was to join a family to help crew a yacht for a week. There was a spare berth, would I like to join them? In ten days time.

Heart in mouth I went to see Miss Yearling, our Superintendent Midwife. She was always kind, and merely said it was time I had a holiday. Ted wrote that in view of the inexperience of the crew a Channel crossing was not contemplated. The first thing I packed was my passport and the first thing he asked when he met me off the train was 'Have you brought your passport?'

The boat was the 'See Otter' based at HMS *Vernon*, Portsmouth. (Now part of Gun Wharf Quays.) 'See Otter' had been one of six German yachts taken as part of war reparations. The skipper, Bruce Davidson, had done the Fastnet Race, but his wife Rosemary did not sail. Their son Peter, 15 years old, was learning fast and his brother Giles, 9 years, was quite handy.

Rosemary and I went off together to shop for provisions and we clicked at once. Sometimes ganged up together against the men…

It was a wonderful week. Our passports were needed. We crossed the Channel to Cherbourg, had several adventures, and, thanks to Bruce and Rosemary, I tried Moules Mariniere. There was a restaurant on the far side of the inner harbour where we were berthed, and they were delighted to find them on the menu. Their enthusiasm for this disgusting looking dish was extraordinary, but when we returned the following evening courage prevailed and I ordered some. Scrumptious. My first ever seafood. It was a good place to start; later on, reading the autobiography of one of the Captains of the *Queen Mary*, he called Cherbourg the seafood capital of the world.

Now, more than sixty years later, I still love seafood. Coincidentally my home is near Oban, The Seafood Capital of Scotland.

Camping holiday

Ted, still in Portsmouth, came to Plymouth on some Naval trip, called to see Maureen and me in our flat, and asked if I would like to join him on a camping trip? Yes, please.

Ted had been a good friend since the early days of the Manadon adventures.

He was short, very good looking and had gorgeous deep blue sailor's eyes. But we were never romantically connected. Just friends, on the same wavelength. So I had no hesitation in saying yes.

With a sailor's skill he stowed all our belongings, camping gear, and two tents onto the back of his scooter and there was still room for me. We headed for Wales, camping for the first night in a field near Cheddar. In the morning Ted bought nearly a pound of Cheddar cheese from the farmer; the best I ever tasted.

We reached the Brecon Beacons, climbed Pen-Y-Fan, survived a lot of rain, enjoyed meals in country pubs, were disappointed with the Sunday morning service we went to in Brecon. Not an interesting service at all, and no Welsh singing!

I chose the start of our route for the return journey, down one of the famous Welsh valleys, finding it gloomy but interesting. Ted was furious. He had NOT come to Wales to see coal mines, heavy industry, waste tips, smoke, railways…

I redeemed myself a bit with a different route through Somerset; he only knew the A38 and thought it a dull county, but he enjoyed the part we rode through, eventually rejoining the A38 much nearer Exeter.

Back at home the aftermath soon became clear. My diary has reminded me that Ted and I had a good, easy chat, agreeing that the expedition had not been 100 per cent successful: 'too much like being married, but not'. Over time I learned by osmosis – in addition to my mother's disgusted fury – that my reputation was gone. No one would believe that our week was platonic. When accepting the invitation I was totally confident that everyone who knew me would know I would 'behave' myself. Any other possible reactions simply did not occur to me. Naivety explains – but does not begin to justify – how, at 23 years old, I could be so stupid.

To make matters worse, a possible, tiny, hint from Ted probably was exactly that – a hint that he hoped for a closer intimacy. Whatever he thought, our friendship gradually petered out.

Once upon a time this sorry tale would have had a moral. But this was 1962; sex was not invented until 1963…. It was only years later I discovered that many of my friends and colleagues had been anticipating 1963 for several years before.

It was tempting to omit this sorry Welsh episode, but it was significant at the time. By the end of 1964 all my friends had married and left

Plymouth. Flatmate Mo had met Alan, another Manadon alumnus, and they were married there in the lovely old tithe barn, recently converted into a charming College chapel. Customary in those days to display wedding presents, theirs were arranged on the billiard table in the Ward Room. Mo's father, who had been an Ordinary Seaman during the war, danced with joy round the table – a very shy man, it was lovely to him so relaxed.

A happy day with Mo and Alan was going to the Helston Floral (Furry) dance. Alan's home was in Helston, so we left Plymouth at 4 am and drove to meet his parents at a flat in the main street. Their friends had invited all of us to their home on the first floor above their shop, which had big windows and gave us a perfect place from which to watch the dancing. As a bride the following year Mo danced in her wedding dress, part of a traditional bride's group.

Meg, who came to share the Connaught Avenue flat after Mo left, had only been with me a month when she met Tony. Manadon again! They too married in the tithe barn chapel.

I had fallen in love with the entire Royal Navy. Not convenient. Not even approved of – it provoked a snide remark from a senior officer's wife that I coveted gold lace on my handbag. She was so wrong. But the town library, unsurprisingly, had a plentiful supply of Naval books both fiction and non-fiction, so RN history and biographies were hoovered up.

Which reminds me that Tony gave Meg, *We Joined the Navy* by John Winton, telling her to read it as it would give her a good idea of naval life. Now, decades later, I still know most of it by heart. And the sequels. And my heart still lifts when all too rarely, a grey ship appears out in the bay. Of course she must be exactly the right shade of grey, not similar ones of visiting foreign Navies here on exercise.

Following Meg's wedding RN contacts were diminishing, an explosion in the birthrate was making the workload in the Maternity Unit stressful and I began to think about pastures new, despite loving Plymouth and originally thinking I was settled there for life.

Departing for Pastures New

One day in February 1965 during a week at home, I took myself up to London for the day. By now both Pat and her sister Liz were in Australia,

Liz writing about midwifery in Sydney. So I went to Australia House to enquire about going out there. After the shortest of waits I saw a man to whom I explained my ideas about wanting to do midwifery, to do it in Sydney, hopefully at the Royal North Shore Hospital. Jovially he replied that if I was as specific as that I could catch the next plane. He sent me off to the New South Wales office, also in The Strand, and there the reaction was much the same. They even gave me the phone number of the Royal North Shore, along with some bumph as well, but having allowed all day for this visit the two offices together took barely ten minutes.

A bit stumped, I stood in The Strand wondering how best to fill in the rest of the day. Something in my brain must have clicked. The City was just down the road, in the City were shipping offices – and nursing at sea was a fashionable pipedream for many at that time. Sue Chapman, of tiddlywinks fame, was actually at sea with Cunard, but not enjoying it much.

A post office was just across the street, so I went in to consult the telephone directories. I stood there trying to think of names of shipping lines, not wanting to go 'bus-stopping' across the Atlantic with Cunard. Worldwide would be more interesting and luckily I thought of P&O. There were four addresses (discovered later that the head office was being rebuilt) and I guessed the medical department was likely to be in the most distant one, which it was.

Middlesex Street, i.e. Petticoat Lane, was hardly recognisable from the famous bustling, jam-packed Sunday street market explored when at King's. There were stalls, but all rather quiet on this weekday morning, so no distractions. I soon found P&O, in a converted factory, and I was directed to the medical department.

A man came to the door and I asked him about possible vacancies, having heard that there was a two-year waiting list. His reply shook me. 'You do realise we get eight applications every day?' I apologised for wasting his time and turned to go, but he asked me to wait a minute and disappeared.

Half an hour later I had been interviewed by the Medical Superintendent, offered a job, and had a medical 'to save me coming up from Plymouth'.

Told I needed to be available at a week's notice, my heart sank. With a Sister's post needing a month's notice, not to mention a flat to pack up and leave, a week was impossible. Not a problem – just write to us when you are ready. Crumbs!

At home, and especially in the hospital, scepticism seemed the main reaction. A Sister named Jeannie Smith was particularly scathing. She had been on the waiting list for ten years but had never heard anything from P&O.

Later on I learnt that all I had done was bypass an initial letter of enquiry. Seeing one was enough to dishearten even the most determined; it had a daunting list of professional requirements: Over the age of 25; SRN; SCM; Operating theatre experience; Private patients experience, and if memory serves me, home nursing too. Scrubbing for Caesars, private wards in all three of my training hospitals, Plymouth; all accepted in my case. This letter ended with a final sentence: 'If ever you are in London please call at this office.' Like many others who thought they were on the waiting list, Jeannie had never done so. All I had done was go straight to the office.

In September I handed in my notice, said goodbye to Plymouth, went home to Oxford and contacted a Nursing Agency. As an Agency midwife I could leave at forty-eight hours notice. I was sent to Abingdon to, believe it or not, the Warren Maternity Home. No rabbits delivered, but a pleasant unit for normal deliveries only. Abingdon is a town full of character, a happy place to be, especially as it was also only a few miles from home.

Chapter 7

P&O Lines SS *Oriana*
1966–1967

ON 4 FEBRUARY 1966 I joined *Oriana* in Southampton.

When getting ready my father gave me an old but unused notebook. It had a lined page, then a blank one, each with the same page number. Hardback, rather flimsy paper, not very interesting, but Daddy thought it might be useful as a supplement to my small, page-a-day diary. Unlikely, I thought, having already been instructed to buy a good camera 'and bring back lots of good photographs'. Slides, in other words, fashionable at the time. As a picture is worth a thousand words the notebook would be *de trop*. By the end of my first voyage it was full. It also started an ever-after custom of writing about special events, particularly holidays.

The diaries were fine for day-to-day doings but more space was welcome for extra long records. What a shock to discover that two outstanding, and exceptional, memories of *Oriana* experiences are nowhere recorded in either diaries or notebooks! Hard to believe that I spent hours trawling for them, without success, hence no specific dates, but photos of the first one are precious.

So are many other photos taken when at sea, including crew and hospital staff. The hospital was well organised, with four wards – one, round a corner and long passage, an isolation ward. Also an operating theatre, pharmacy, outpatients waiting room, small kitchen, sluice etc., not to mention two lock-up padded cells. It was staffed by a surgeon, assistant surgeon, three nursing sisters, a busy pharmacist and two male orderlies. Too many reminiscences about our work and play to embark on here!

The background to the first outstanding memory is historical. *Oriana* was built to be the flagship of the Orient Line, but early in 1960 – within weeks of being launched in November 1959 by Princess Alexandra – the Orient Line had been taken over by P&O. However *Oriana* continued to sail under the Orient Line house flag, and many of her crew had been with the Orient Line for the whole of their careers.

The first shock was the arrival of a new Commodore – a P&O man! The first in this ship, and as the two lines had different traditions there was much angst among the old hands. *Oriana* sailed on. Rumours began to spread.

The Commodore was visiting the engine room. and other departments, at 6 am! The Commodore had been to see the Chinese laundry men at the laundry in the bowels of the ship. Unheard of! Why are the nursing sisters not wearing their caps? Some quick thinking man replied that in this ship only the sister on duty wore her cap. The reply was accepted. The new boss was quiet, calm, not seeking trouble, just getting to know his ship. The crew settled down. One day in the middle of the Pacific, a signal arrived, saying the Orient Line house flag was to be lowered immediately and the P&O house flag raised. Six years after her launch, *Oriana* was now to be visibly part of P&O. Of course the news went round the ship like lightning; cue for great unhappiness in many of the crew. A main bone of contention was *why now? in the middle of a voyage?* Watch this space… .

Both constraint of duties and narrow accommodation meant that no parties or other events were ever held in the senior officers 'alleyway'. Suddenly, all officers not on duty were invited up there. At lunch time. On arrival we were greeted by the Purser and Chief Engineer wearing black top hats and black arm bands, handing us glasses of Black Velvet. Chopin's Funeral March played in the background – sombre tones never heard on board. Then we were led to pay our salaams to the deceased. Blocking the alleyway was a coffin, draped in an Orient Line flag and topped with a wreath.

The wake did not last long, but doubtless memorable for everyone, certainly never forgotten by me. Once again news travelled at high speed all round the ship, honour was satisfied and there was never another word of complaint. The Commodore, tactfully, had been missing, but the Staff Captain was host and chief mourner, proof that officialdom had listened. Many times I have told this as a perfect example of excellent man-management.

The second tale concerns a passenger. P&O company policy was for off duty officers to socialise with passengers. (Cunard policy was rigid separation.)

One evening our first class hostess gave a small drinks party in her cabin for Cary Grant, who had joined the ship in Los Angeles with his wife Dyan and 10-month-old daughter, Jennifer, for the voyage home to England. After an evening surgery in the hospital I was the last to arrive. The cabin was small and crowded, and I was soon in the middle of the crush, but with no one to talk to. Suddenly standing next to Cary, he began explaining his theory that as he was an older dad his daughter would benefit from his life experience, and be a calm and contented baby.

We had not been introduced, but standing close to his group I felt emboldened to join in, explaining that my father was 47 when my sister was born, but she certainly was not a calm and contented baby. Cary was 65 so probably regarded 47 as youthful. Anyhow my disagreement was taken in good part, but I was so shocked at my cheek I have never remembered Cary's exact reply – though think we agreed to disagree. Nor do I remember anything of the rest of the party.

Perhaps not as drastic as arguing with a Matron but it could have caused an unwise upset. I do remember that some of us were friendly with the baby's nanny, who confirmed that she was indeed a calm and contented baby. Anyway there was no unfortunate repercussion, and at the end of the voyage Cary presented the Purser with a gold watch, thanking him for a comfortable voyage.

It was well earned apparently, as the list of requirements sent pre-voyage, had been mind- boggling and headache making. Presentations were not something that always happened, since we heard via the grapevine that the Grant family return voyage in a different P&O ship provoked a very different reaction…

Many tales were written about shore excursions, but this book must try not to become a travelogue. Any member of the crew not on Watch was permitted to join any excursion if a seat was available, but always on the understanding that a written report might be required.

One vastly different tale is another favourite, and one beloved of the crew. Years before, a cargo ship had a much loved Chief Engineer who died suddenly. Not wishing to bury him at sea, he was dressed in his white tropical uniform and put into a refrigeration unit to be taken home to England. Shortly afterwards, in the hottest part of the Red Sea, the ship broke down. The fault could not be traced and the ship wallowed in the heat for many hours, to the despair of the engineers.

Suddenly, on the top-level grating of the engine room, the Chief appeared, looking down in his usual calm way and as always with his usual small hammer in his hand, and a bundle of cotton waste. Shortly afterwards the fault was found, rectified, and the ship resumed her voyage home. On arrival the Chief's compartment was opened with some trepidation. Would he be there? Yes he was; looking as serene as ever and with his white uniform as immaculate as when put on. Except that there was oil on the soles of his socks...

Mariners have a lovely custom of welcoming other mariners on board their ship whenever or wherever they are in port. One evening in Hong Kong the deputy surgeon, the pharmacist and I went ashore to do a tour of a typhoon shelter. In the shelters a whole community existed, with entire lives being spent on board junks. Sampans could be hired for visitors to be rowed through the 'streets', apparently welcome to see all aspects of lives on board. Families eating meals, musical instruments being played, children playing, girls in gaudy costumes sitting alone on the rear deck of their vessel, with a red light hanging above them...

Back at the quay as we disembarked, a very pretty little Chinese girl, who looked not more than 14 years old, approached the boys. I have never seen more horrified men, and they rushed me off at speed to find a taxi. At the Ocean Terminal a small Chinese passenger liner was berthed on the other side from *Oriana*. It was nearing midnight, everywhere was quiet, and I decided now was the time to test the universal mariners' welcome. Once again the boys were unhappy, but I marched across the brow to the entrance, to be given a pleasant welcome by the guard, in rather fractured English. The surgeon was ashore he said, but if we could come back tomorrow afternoon we could meet her. Next afternoon Angus, the assistant surgeon and I were on duty, but we had no inpatients in the hospital. so I rang the teleops to tell them if there were any calls for us we were on the other side of the terminal in the Chinese ship. There was rather a shocked reaction but as long as we were in the vicinity and our whereabouts known there were no rules broken.

Once again we were welcomed, and this time the surgeon was called and she took us on a brief tour of the public rooms of the ship before taking us to her medical department.

We were given Russian champagne and Russian chocolate; discussed various things including pay – the surgeon earned the equivalent of my nursing sister's salary; and then she and Angus began a professional chat. She was concerned about the First Officer, who she felt sure had a duodenal ulcer but he refused to believe her. It seemed his career would be threatened. Angus was ready to see him if he would agree, so he was sent for, and a tall, spare, grey haired man came in. I treasure a memory of the British and Chinese doctors prodding his tummy together and and with no hesitation Angus corroborated her diagnosis. It was a most classic duodenal ulcer. We were so sorry for the patient, another pleasant member of the crew, but at least one hoped he was glad to have a second opinion – even though it confirmed his fear for the future.

After our happy afternoon next door I rang to tell the teleops we were back, and got the impression they were very relieved, having imagined us being arrested or abducted or suffering some other drastic fate.

By the end of fifteen months in *Oriana* there was every chance that on arrival in Southampton I would be told to join another ship. Tales of the other eleven passenger liners were not very beguiling, also too long at sea was not wise for a career, especially midwifery. (There was an unexpected delivery on board one day, but unfortunately I was at lunch.) With much sadness I left, having enjoyed five long voyages and one cruise.

The first and last long ones were from Southampton to Australia and New Zealand, then across the Pacific to Canada via Fiji and Honolulu. From Vancouver to San Francisco and Los Angeles before recrossing the Pacific, to Japan, Hong Kong and Singapore prior to returning home the way we came – via Aden and the Mediterranean. Two more voyages circumnavigated the globe; one West to East, the other East to West. The fifth one was out to Australia and NZ, to Honolulu again and the west coast of America, then returning home via the same ports. The cruise was a fortnight to the Mediterranean.

How privileged I was! How lucky! My red Seaman's Card is still a treasure.

Chapter 8

Domiciliary Midwife Liverpool

1967–1972

THE NEXT FIVE years were not the easiest, but of course included some varied episodes, including one in Odiham, via Mrs Gardiner's Nursing Agency, where I spent three rather sad months in the cottage hospital while working out a permanent decision. Matron was an unhappy person , home from a job in London she had loved, now resentfully somewhat housebound caring for a very elderly mother. Her ire included all of us and made for some odd difficulties.

The hospital itself was delightful, still regarded by the locals as their own even after twenty years of the NHS. Eggs and other gifts still arrived, and as a new member of staff I was invited to sherry one day with two elderly ladies, stalwarts of the village. At 11 am. A traditional 'sherry time' in decades past. They were charming, and it was a relaxed and happy visit to their pretty cottage in the main street, despite only having met once before. Nevertheless a surprise was in store; astonishing to discover they were aunts of David Attenborough, famous even in 1967. Such name dropping. What fun!

From three months in Odiham, I returned to The Warren in Abingdon, again via the agency, as it transpired I could resume practising midwifery at once as long as I did a mandatory refresher course ASAP. I loved Abingdon, a town full of character, but for some reason staying there was not an option.

I had begun 1967 as a nursing sister on *Oriana*, and ended it as a district midwife in Liverpool. I was 31 years old, had to earn my own living but had no ambitions or plans for a career in midwifery nor realistic thoughts about any alternatives. However, as one of those rare midwives who enjoyed both hospital and home deliveries, but not district nursing or health visiting, a city post was necessary. A country post combined all three. Liverpool seemed a good choice, but I had not asked the right professional questions, largely just thinking of it as a good place for exploring the north of England when off-duty. Not so, too far in any direction to get to really interesting areas.

Due to the increasing birth-rate Bradford had recently introduced forty-eighty hour discharges, to release the pressure on hospitals. Following normal deliveries, and all being well, the mums and babies went home to the care of district midwives for the remainder of the ten days they would normally have stayed in hospital. Another newish practice in some places was for district midwives to deliver their patients in hospital and take them home soon afterwards.

None of these new ideas were ever going to happen in Liverpool, but I was poor at interviews, never thinking it could be reasonable to ask questions for myself, only answer those put to me.

Liverpool had excellent maternity hospitals, and it also had a dwindling population as many citizens were rehoused in new towns like Skelmersdale and Runcorn, as well as new council estates on the outskirts of the city. There were beds available for any woman who wished to be delivered in hospital. Added to that, midwives would never be allowed to deliver their patients in hospital, as I learnt not long before leaving. Apparently there was 'War at the top', with no cooperation between the two department heads responsible.

The midwives' house in West Derby was passed on to me by a very nice girl who was leaving to get married. Down the road from West Derby village, with an old stone wall edging Lord Sefton's estate at the bottom of the garden, with fields beyond, it was part of a post-war new-build area, an end of terrace house, and very comfortable. The City Council looked after us well.

A pupil midwife would spend three months with me, (not residential) needing to do three home deliveries in that time. Hard to believe, but towards the end of my four years we would be sent miles beyond my own district to anywhere in the city, in order to achieve the required three, thanks to the dwindling population mentioned.

My first pupil was a lovely middle-aged Irish Roman Catholic nun. She had belonged to her Order since she was 18 years old, always nursing or teaching. Now she was to go home to Ireland as a Matron and Mother Superior, so needed to complete her midwifery qualification by doing Part II of her training. She adored the babies and loved going into people's homes.

When she left she gave me a beautiful little white nylon bedjacket. It had small frills round all the edges and pink rosebuds round the neck and is still one of my treasures. After finishing her three months with me she was going to the Mother House of her Order, in Bowden, Cheshire. I was starting a week's leave and offered to drive her over there.

On arriving we walked into a celebration. Earlier that day a young nun had made her final vows and the celebratory evening meal included an iced wedding cake as she was now, as I understand, a bride of Christ. It was a happy, most enjoyable evening. There were only a few nuns, perhaps nine or ten. They ran a small hospital, actually a care home for the elderly. At 9 pm I started to say goodbye, ready to drive back to Liverpool, but they were horrified. It was far too late and of course I must stay the night. My assurances about driving home unavailing.

I had been shown the chapel – and some beautiful vestments – and learnt that they had a service every morning at 7.30 am. Tentatively I suggested that I would like to join them, but instantly, and hilariously, I was turned down. 'Indeed you will not! They will say we are trying to convert you! You will stay in your bed and we will bring your breakfast.'

Escorted to a very comfortable bedroom, I found every conceivable thing provided for an unexpected stay. Nightdress, dressing gown, slippers, toiletries etc., even a packet of 'bunnies' (sanitary towels), which were very welcome. After an excellent sleep the door opened next morning at 8 am. Two nuns came in carrying an enormous, laden wooden tray. The works. Huge cooked breakfast, plus fruit juice, cereal, toast, butter and marmalade, coffee…

When saying goodbye they gave me an envelope. Inside were two white handkerchiefs with tatting lace round the edges and a big triangular insert in one corner. Beautiful. A note with them said they were a wee memento of Bowden. Another incredible episode for my memory scrapbook, and two more treasures.

Early one morning, for some reason without a pupil, I delivered a baby in Aintree. About to take a bowl of water to mum I managed instead to throw it all over the kitchen floor. I was mortified and apologetic, but Dad said at once: 'You're all right nurse', in his rich Scouse accent, a perfect example of the kindness of Liverpudlians. Driving home afterwards at 6 am I crossed Aintree Racecourse along the Melling Road. It was a glorious morning and it was Grand National Day, but although the car windows were open there was not a sound, except for a blackbird singing. Yet another entry for the memory scrapbook.

For much of those years I had a companion, a much-loved black and white cat. He came to me as a half-grown kitten after I answered an advert on the Post Office door. The following weekend was my once-a-month four days off, when almost always I went home to Oxford. Telling my sister about the new kitten, and concerned about what to do with him, she said to bring him with me. Which is how he learnt to commute up and down the M6 etc,. rapidly being at home at either end of the journey and quickly recognising when we were nearly there. It was also during that first weekend that he learnt his name.

The day he came to me happened to be my parents' Coral wedding anniversary. During my *Oriana* days the ship had visited Fiji, and from Suva, along with many others, I was delighted to take home chunks of Fijian coral. They were often sold in wide, flat, plaited-palm baskets, sometimes hideously dyed in violent pink, yellow or purple colours. Seeing them growing, through trips in glass-bottomed boats, was brilliant. Much better, but no thoughts of environmental damage in those days. A great tradition when the ship sailed was a musical farewell on the quay played by the police band. They had very smart and unforgettable uniforms – black jackets with white mid-calf length skirts ending in serrated hems.

The Coral wedding coincidence, and black and white uniforms, suggested Suva for the kitten's name. My father was so taken with the idea he spent the whole weekend calling Suva, and by the time we went home the black and white bundle of fur always responded to his name. Parting with him when I left Liverpool was a dreadful wrench.

My time in Liverpool ended abruptly, after a visitor to my door was the final straw. An acquaintance of mine died and between this and her funeral, her husband turned up on my doorstep carrying a bundle of newspapers (I collected them for charity, coordinated by the local scout troop). He gave them to me then to my horror, flung his arms around me and wanted to take me out to dinner. One difficult episode too many. I slammed the door, burst into tears and resigned next day.

What next? Something radical needed.

Chapter 9

Mrs Gardiner's Nursing Agency QARNNS

1971–1972

FOR A THIRD time I contacted Mrs Gardiner's Nursing Agency in Caversham.

Mrs Gardiner happened to be in Wallasey. She came over to Liverpool and took me to the Adelphi, the city's poshest hotel, for coffee. We talked for over an hour – well, she did, about her work.

By then I had contacted the Royal Navy, had an advisory interview, filled in forms, posted certificates and been given an interview date.

The agency gave me a choice of four home nursing jobs. Three sounded impossible, demanding beyond belief, so it was a simple choice to go to a farm in Wiltshire. The farmer, Mr Swanton, was about to be discharged from the local hospital.

Asked to arrive the evening before, I was given a warm welcome by his extremely pleasant wife. Next morning the ambulance drove in to the courtyard, the doors opened – and I was horrified. In front of me was a frail and very ill old man, not the vigorous and difficult patient I had been told to expect. Convinced he was about to leave this world, he did, less than forty-eight hours later. I was really upset; even after such a short time feeling part of the household. No more private home nursing for me.

When I rang the agency with the news Mrs Gardiner spoke to me herself. She asked me to think about giving up the Navy idea and become her assistant. First I went to Wisbech Hospital for a month in the

New student nurse set. August 1953 WMOH (Wingfield Morris Orthopaedic Hospital).

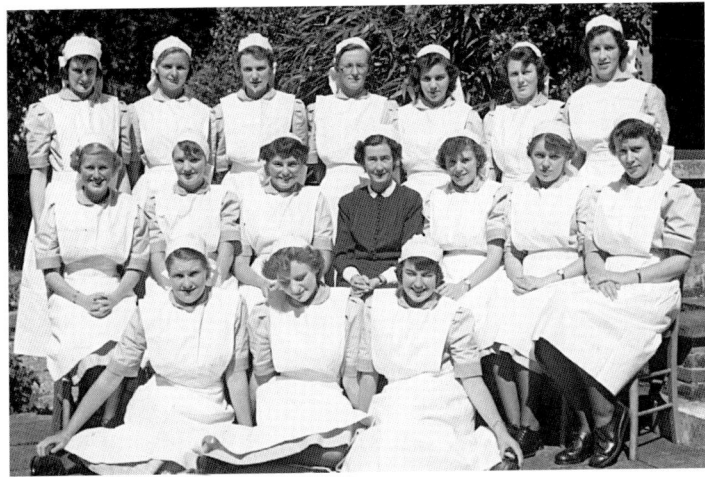

Right: Student nurse WMOH.

Far right: Third year student nurse in 'Kipper' cap. KCH (King's College Hospital)

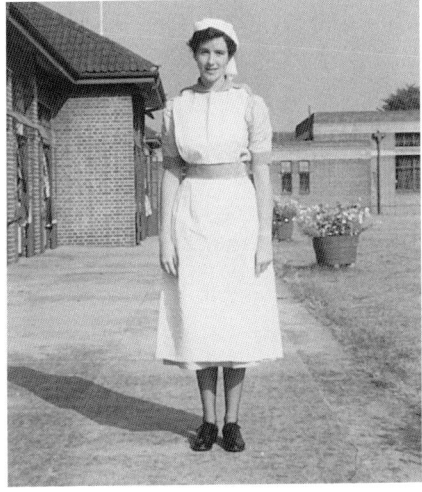

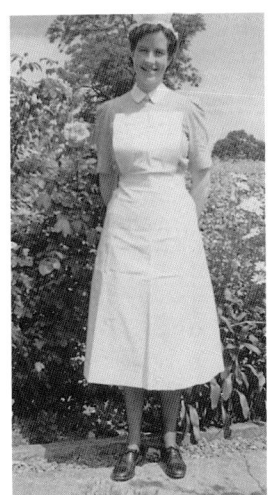

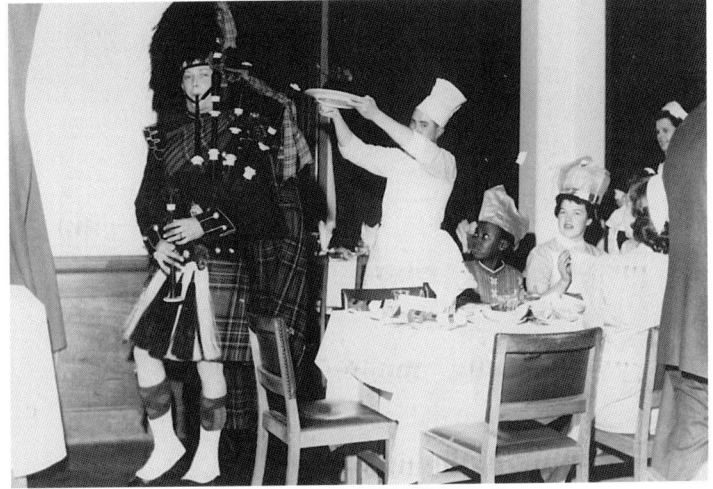

Nurses' Christmas dinner KCH 1955.

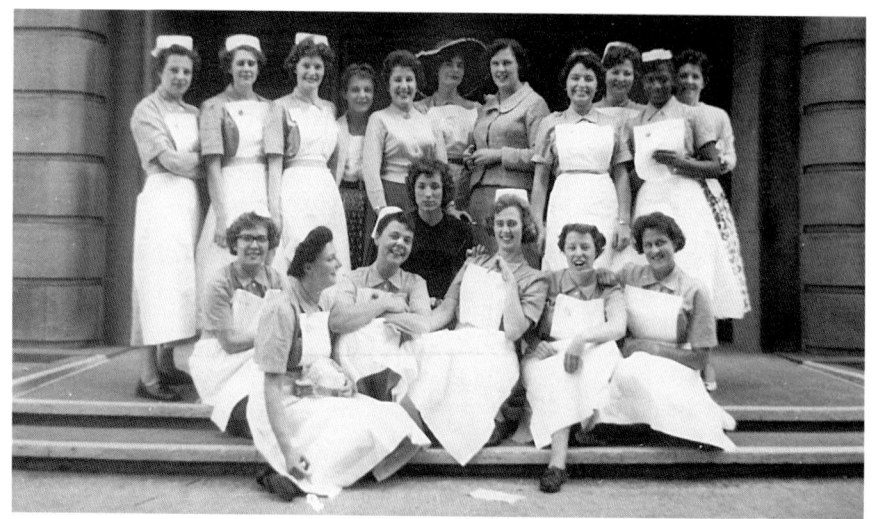

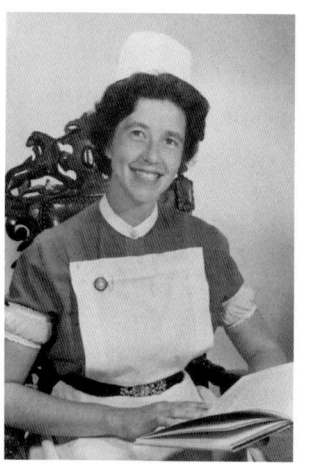

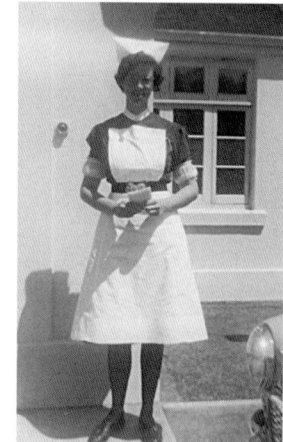

Above: Pupil midwives. February 1959 set. QCMH (Queen Charlotte's Maternity Hospital).

Far left: Staff midwife FFH (Freedom Fields Hospital Plymouth).

Left: Midwifery Sister DMH (Devonport Maternity Home).

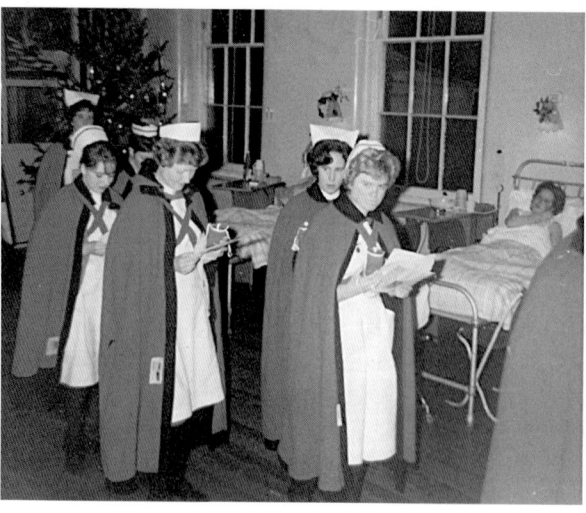

Christmas Eve Carol singing round wards DMH.

Right: Heros ½ beached on Drake's Island Plymouth Sound. Jenny, Ted, Tony, hauling.

Below left: Hospital staff P&O Lines SS *Oriana* 1966.

Below right: 'Funeral' of Orient Line House flag. P&O *Oriana* in the Pacific.

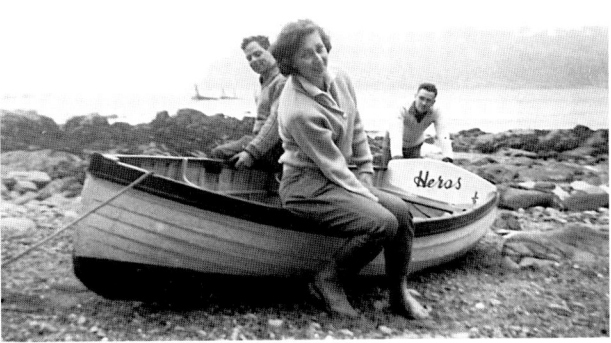

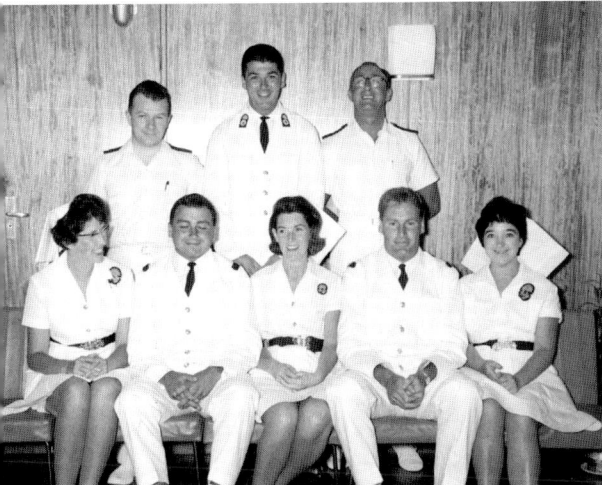

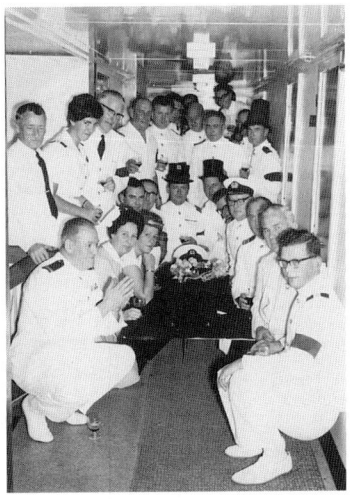

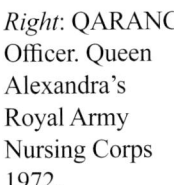

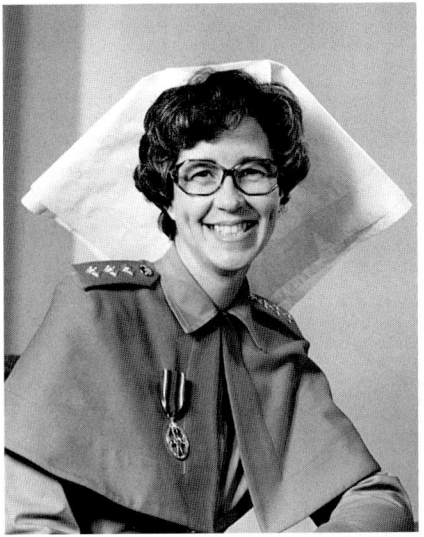

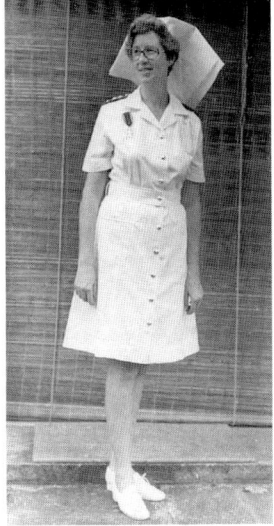

Right: QARANC Officer. Queen Alexandra's Royal Army Nursing Corps 1972.

Far right: QA Tropical uniform.

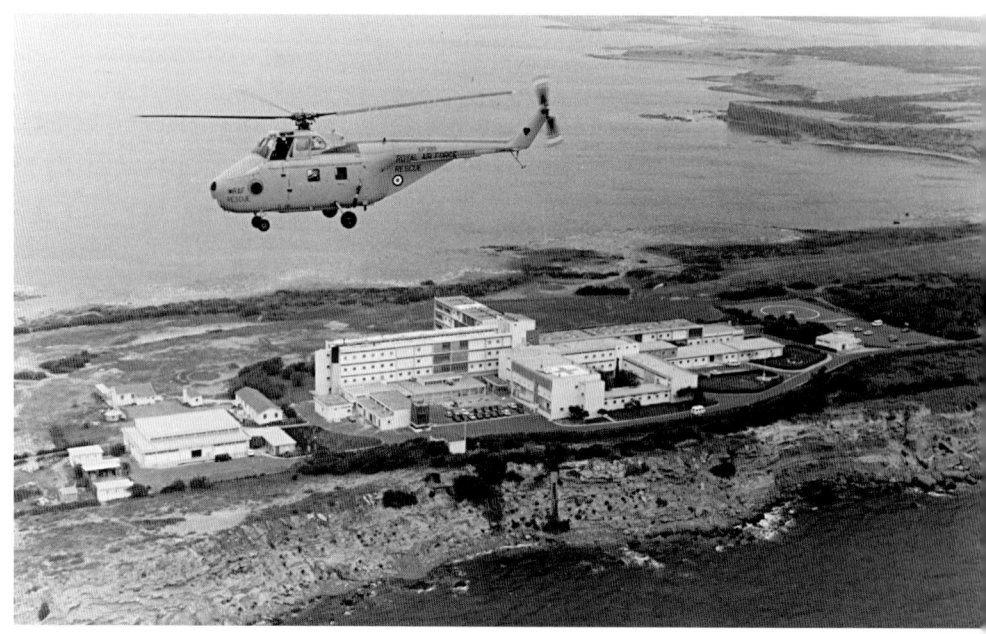

TPMH (The Princess Mary's Hospital RAF Akrotiri). (UK MOD)

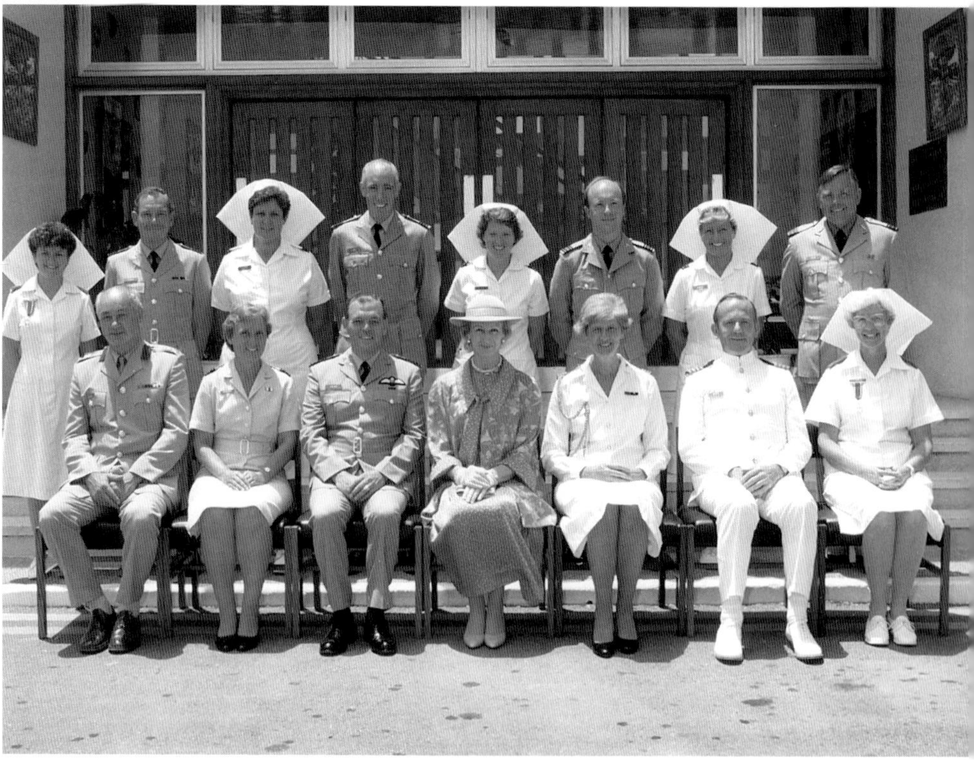

HRH Princess Alexandra, Patron PMRAFNS, with Hospital staff TPMH 1987. (UK MOD)

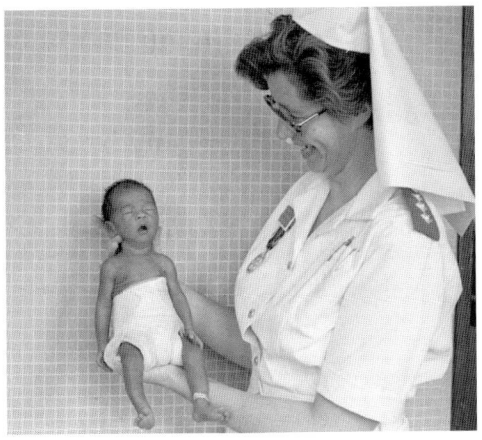 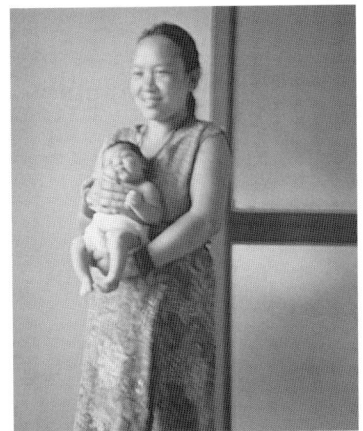

Above left: QA midwife with Gurkha baby BMH British Military Hospital Hong Kong.

Above right: Gurkha 'Didi' (woman) with her baby. BMH Dharan Nepal.

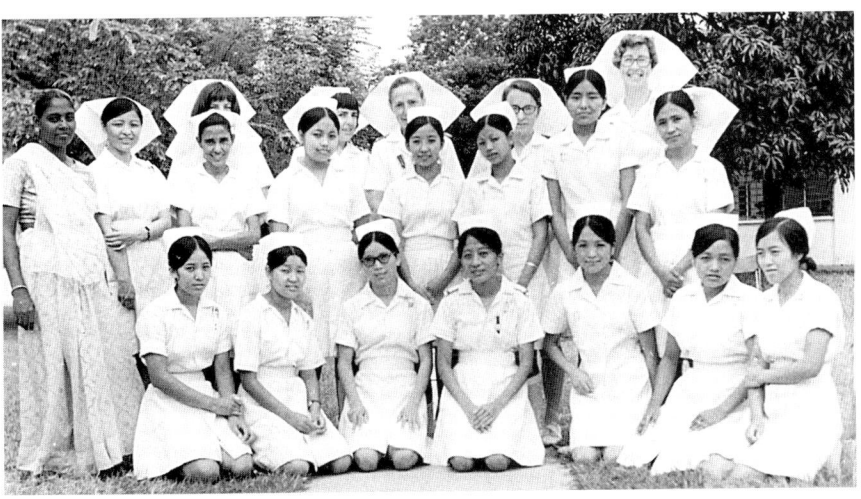

Above: Nursing Staff BMH Dharan Nepal.

Right: QA staff BMH Berlin.

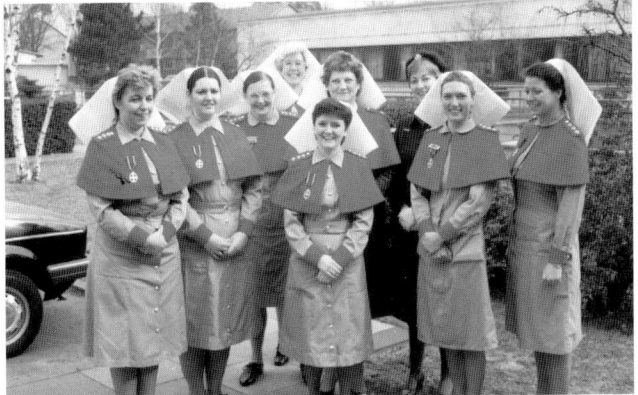

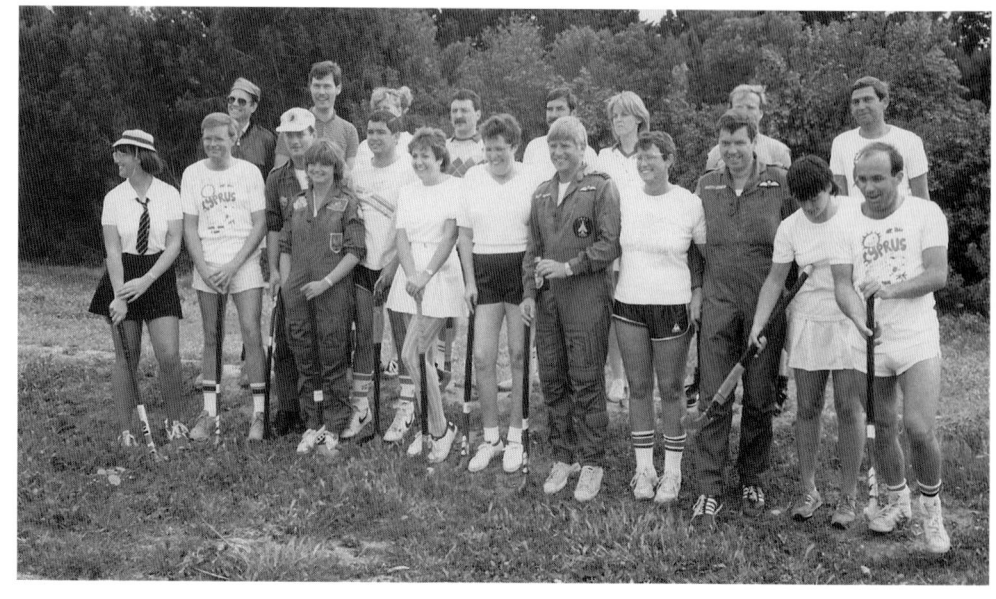

Hockey teams TPMH and 5 Squadron RAF Akrotiri.

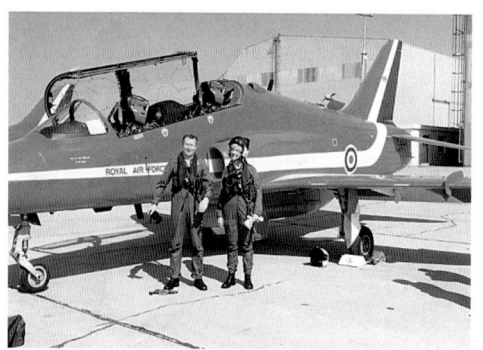

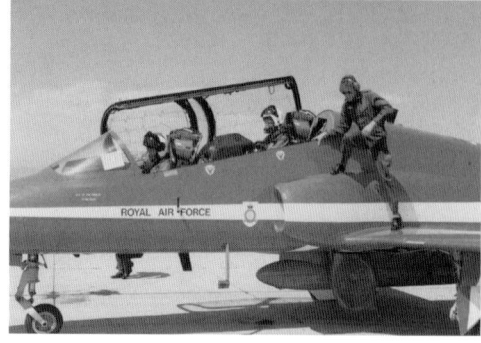

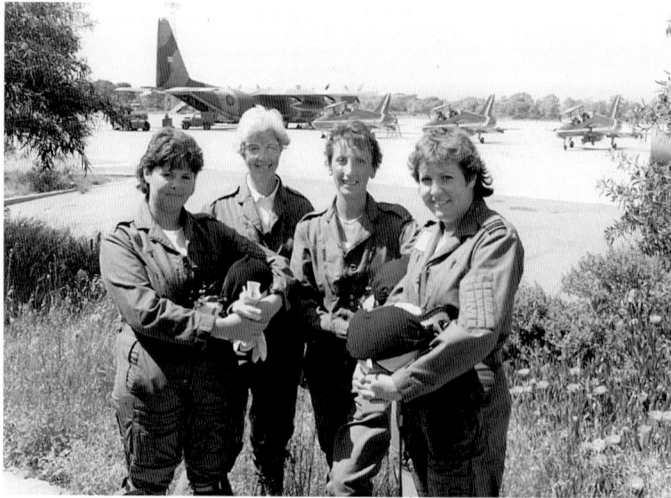

Above left: Red Arrow Pilot with passenger RAF Akrotiri.

Above right: Preparing for take-off.

Left: One QA, three PMs equipped for Red Arrow flights.

Red Arrows Bomb
Blast formation.

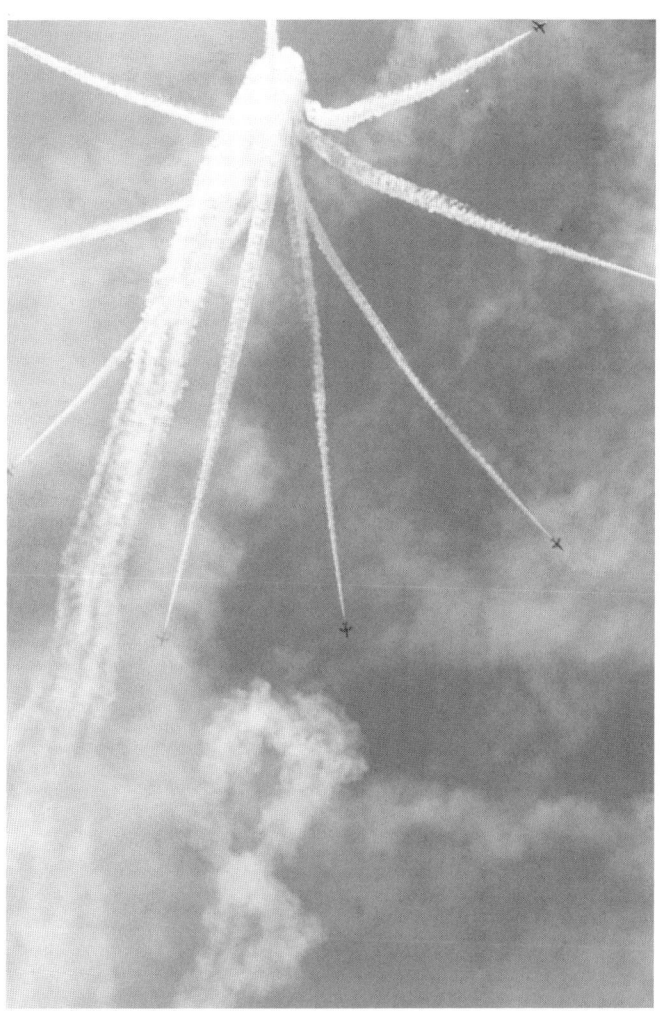

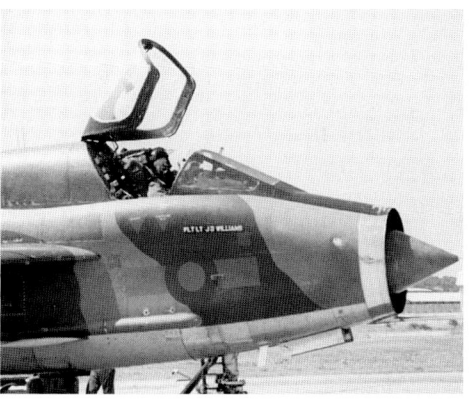
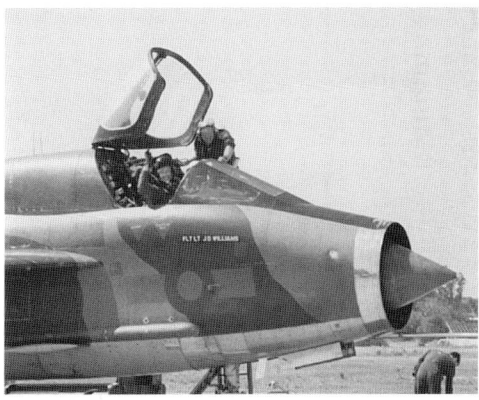

Above left: Passenger, RAF Lightning aircraft RAF Akrotiri.

Above right: Preparing for Lightning take-off RAF Akrotiri.

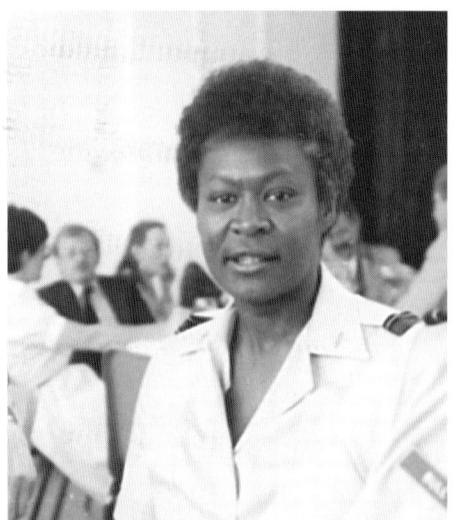
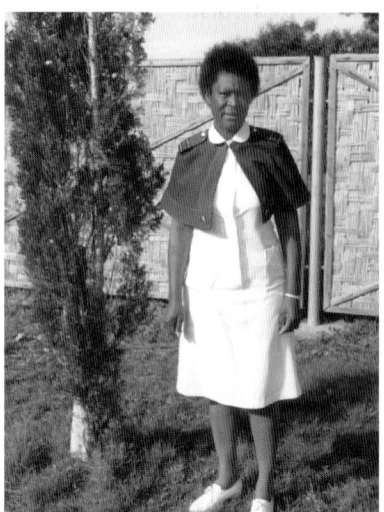

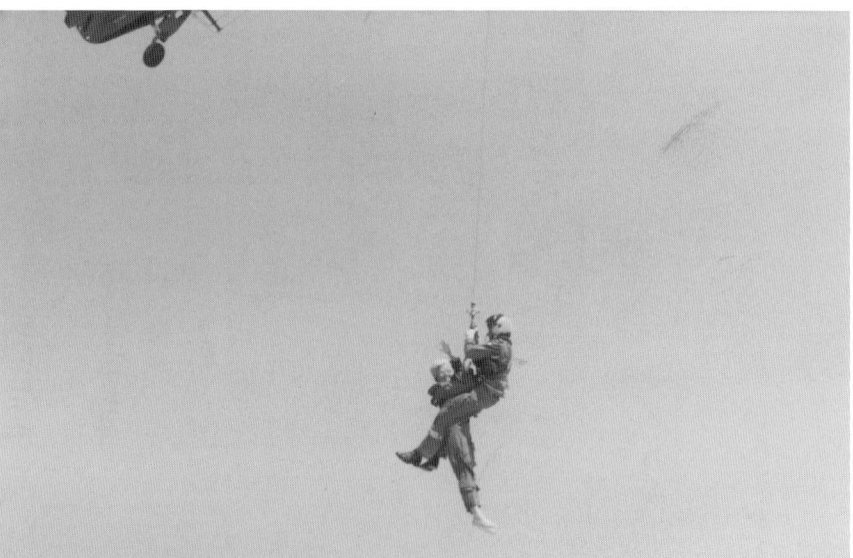

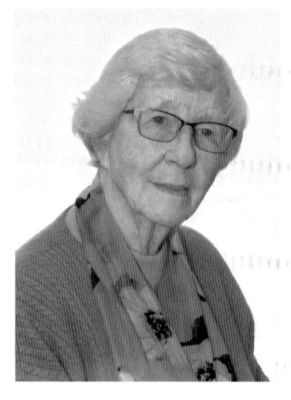

Top left: Squadron Leader Yvonne Mapp TPMRAFNS. A special friend and support.

Top right: Yvonne Mapp. Disliked facing a camera.

Above: Air/sea rescue. Landing craft to helicopter at sea off Akrotiri Peninsula.

Left: Lady Africa Commission Mary Sandilands 2023 Author Never Argue With A Matron.

maternity unit, using all my off duty for interesting explorations of East Anglia, not least Sandringham. The church there was incredible, a small, ordinary country church from the outside, inside awash with ornate furnishings, including a silver altar. The rector appeared, and kindly showed me more treasures, especially a huge Bible with a silver cover – I think I remember it being inset with gem stones. It had belonged to Queen Alexandra.

On completion of the month in Wisbech I joined the Agency in Caversham, across the bridge over the Thames from Reading. Mrs Gardiner had found a flat for me, and I have 'dined out' on my first night there ever since. The house looked like an ordinary Victorian two storey end of terrace one, near the town centre. Two flats on the first and second floors were occupied by several girls. My flat was an odd conversion of what had been an attic. The internal living area was accessed only by a short flight of steps just hidden by a curtain, inside the second floor flat. No door.

It was a narrow gallery, lit by a big skylight, surrounding an empty space; presumably the ceiling of the room below. Into this had been fitted around the sides a linear arrangement of cooker, sink, shower, a table and two small armchairs. A door into a very large bedroom was in the far corner of this set up. Now, please pay attention to the layout in there...

Just inside, to the left of the door stood an enormous mahogany wardrobe, which partly concealed the single bed along the same wall beyond it. Diagonally across the room from the door stood another single bed, at a right angle to the concealed one.

I moved in without meeting any of my neighbours, settled in, and chose the bed behind the wardrobe. About 3 am I woke up when the light was switched on and saw two men walking in. Luckily always instantly fully awake, I sat up, bed clothes chastely pulled round my shoulders, and told them to get out, having guessed at once what had happened.

'Oh, it's quite all right,' one reassured me. '------ told us we could stay here.'

'I have taken this flat, and no one else is staying here. Leave NOW!'

Realisation dawned that someone was already in the room. The first young blood turned and came over to me, holding out his hand and saying in a cut glass accent 'Hello, I'm Ralph.' His companion clearly thought this was the polite thing to do so he came over too, holding out his hand and saying 'Hello, I'm Nigel.'

Desperate not to laugh, at last I convinced them they were NOT staying. and they left. Next evening when I got back to the flat I was met by four frightened and contrite girls, certain I would complain to the landlady. Of course, they had not known that the new tenant had moved in. The party they all went to ended much later than expected, so they told the two boys they could stay in the room upstairs, exactly as I had guessed. It took quite a while to assure them that I had no intention of telling the landlady, and even longer to convince them that I thought it hilarious. In fact I had a suspicion they regarded me as a bit odd for finding Nigel and Ralph so amusing.

Although flattered by Mrs Gardiner's offer, and in many ways enjoying helping to run the Agency, I decided against accepting. Four of us manned the telephone, in close proximity in one office. A happy group, until her deputy picked on me, and nothing I could do was right; she was most unpleasant to me. Apparently I was not her first victim; she had form, as Mrs Gardiner was aware

Queen Alexandra's Royal Naval Nursing Service

Having fallen in love with the entire Royal Navy in Plymouth, nevertheless I could not see myself nursing in the RN. However, as said, something drastic needed to be done after leaving Liverpool, and one day in the city I went into the RN Recruiting Office, which was a bad start. As a qualified nurse, therefore potential officer, I should have applied via one of the frequent advertisements in the Nursing Journals. Recruiting offices were for other ranks.

Not that anyone ever said so, but the underlying implication was there. Eventually I was given a date for interview, several months ahead, December 1971, in the Empress State Building in West London.

The interview was a bit daunting. The Matron in Chief was austere, cool and formal. I did not take to her, and doubt she took to me. She certainly disapproved of the rather jolly approach of her male colleague, a Commodore. He asked if I met the Navy in Plymouth...

An obvious question, which I expected, was how would I feel about working with younger people who would be senior to me, and after having my own house how would I feel living in a Mess?

After the interview Matron's friendly secretary, who shepherded each applicant, asked, in an almost off-hand way, why I wanted to join the Navy. She loved my answer, but with hindsight strongly suspect it would not have amused the MIC. I told about the group of noisy lads on the Friday afternoon train from Helensburgh to Glasgow, and how a drunken young sailor had insisted they 'Shush' because there was a Lady present. He made me realise – again – how much I loved the Navy, but it could not be called a serious or tactful reason.

The Navy only had a tiny midwifery branch, and with Malta closed probably had more than enough midwives. Dom Mintoff, the Maltese Prime Minister, had recently forced the Royal Navy to abandon its base in Malta, which had been the busy and much-loved home of the British Mediterranean Fleet for centuries.

In fact I was at Freedom Fields when a Medical Branch Commander was sent to us to brush up his obstetrics, before taking charge of the new branch. Previously the Royal Navy ignored the existence of Naval wives, unlike the Army which had looked after them for more than a century. We also had a Registrar for two years, a very efficient doctor who was a Naval officer, probably destined to be the hands-on obstetrician while the Commander did admin. After leaving Freedom Fields I never heard of either of them again.

My interview included a very good Christmas lunch in the canteen, enjoyed with the other five hopeful applicants, then a rigorous medical. The equipment for eye testing was outstanding, far more impressive than anything I ever saw at the Royal Eye Hospital or anywhere else. It has remained an indelible memory.

The six of us who met that day had kept in touch, just to share our fates. Only one was accepted. The letter turning me down was at the flat at 1am when I returned after an evening baby-sitting the Agency phones. (We provided a twenty-four hour service.) I burst into tears, went to bed, slept well, and got up next morning deciding that I would interview the Army.

Later, I learnt that the QA's, and RAF nurses, were all subject to the Army, or RAF, Discipline Acts, but the QARNNS retained a quasi-civilian status.

They were proud of 'not needing' to be subject to Naval Discipline, being too ladylike. I think this distinction played a part at the Naval interview, and also I noticed it as a subtle attitude when visiting Naval sisters. In Hong Kong one of them became a friend when she came to spend one day a week in our Special Care baby unit 'to keep her hand in'. Back in the UK she invited me to visit her, in the large, lovely old Royal Naval Hospital in Gosport. It was enlightening to see her on duty. She appeared to be a figurehead only, not at all hands-on, with her sailor male nurses doing all the work, and being noticeably deferential. She was an officer, of course, but so were the QAs and PMs, and I like to think that rank was less important to us when on duty. We worked as a team.

Having interviewed the Army (!) and been impressed, it was cheering to receive an acceptance letter.

Chapter 10

Queen Alexandra's Royal Army Nursing Corps

1972–2001

ON THE ORIGINAL application form one had to state whether prepared to stay two years – the minimum – four years, or eight. Needing to settle, and determined to cope, I ticked eight. At interview I was persuaded to reduce to four; there seemed doubt that anyone had ever opted for eight. I stayed nineteen years. Mandatory retirement for Majors, at 55 years old, ended my QA days.

On 1 May 1972 I reported to Aldershot, to start my life in the Corps – with a badly swollen ankle strongly strapped up. Not best for marching. Luckily we spent minimal time on the parade square. The damage had happened in Banbury when crossing the road from the hospital, where I worked for three weeks while waiting to join the Corps. After traffic had passed I set off – but left one foot stuck in a pothole. My ankle soon blew up like a balloon, and after hobbling over to the Sisters' home I was taken to casualty. A very experienced Polish doctor strapped it up, and gave me some excellent advice. Not least that it would continue to swell to some extent for a year, which it did.

QATC

The QA Training Centre was at the Royal Pavilion in Aldershot, though not the one built for Queen Victoria. That had been a wooden chalet, erected in 1855 on a site chosen by Prince Albert, for Her Majesty to use when she went to review her troops.

When I joined, the chalet had been replaced by a series of modern concrete blocks built on the same site, but still set in extensive and beautiful grounds. From the main gate a long drive wound up to the Officers' Mess, lined by dozens of rhododendrons which blazed with colour when in bloom. A great variety of trees, and wide lawns, added to the grandeur, and close to the Mess was a monkey puzzle tree said to have been planted by Prince Albert.

The new buildings were not quite Brutalist architecture, but the flat roof leaked, and it was very cold inside. However, the rooms were spacious and the furniture comfortable. One year when I was there a nightingale sang night after night in the thick hedgerow opposite my room.

Our basic training lasted just three weeks, and there were only seven of us new recruits. After five years of being cajoled to 'Make love, not war', joining the armed forces was deeply unfashionable.

We were the despair of the experienced male sergeant who tried to teach us to march. One girl was so short she could not manage the regulation twenty-seven inch step, another never overcame marching Dutch doll style, with an arm and leg swinging forward on the same side, most amusing to watch but not conducive to Good Order and Discipline.

I was the only one with a car, and most days drove into town with people wanting lifts. The centre was often full of squaddies, and they had to salute us. We of course, had to return their salutes, but I was nervous and used to creep along hoping not to encounter any of them. A happy discovery was finding that any talk or discussion about the Royal Family was welcome. The King is the ultimate boss of everyone in the Armed Forces (though then, of course, it was the Queen).

At the end of our three weeks the others had organised a surprise. They gave me a pretty blue Jasper Wedgwood box, together with a card pronouncing me an Honorary Member of the Royal Corps of Transport! In today's fully integrated services, no one would believe that we were given just one morning learning about the 'Big Army' as we called it. I remember nothing about it, other than being taken to the RAMC Training Centre (Royal Army Medical Corps) and shown a large table with a potential battle plan layout. Presumably we were given some explanations about various units etc., especially medical ones.

Another unimaginable note today is that we were assumed to be Ladies. Not so in the WRAC (Womens' Royal Army Corps), the forerunner of which had been the wartime Auxiliary Territorial Service. In their basic training they were taught etiquette; how to be ladylike; and among other things, flower arranging.

Louise Margaret Maternity Hospital

My first posting was not much more than a mile from the Training Centre, to another Victorian foundation, Louise Margaret Maternity Hospital. This time the original hundred-year-old building was still in use, sitting at the far end of the enormous Cambridge Military Hospital, on top of a long hill above the town.

All newly joined midwives were sent to LMMH first. Military obstetric practices proved to be excellent, probably for two reasons.

During the years after the war the RAMC had been concentrating on improving the standard of the Medical Services, then recently the Director had been an obstetric and gynaecology specialist. Soon after going to LMMH it dawned on me that in my mind I had always worked *with* doctors, but, after almost twenty years, I now realised that doctors regarded nurses and midwives as working *for* them. Handmaids had become nursemaids, not a helpful analogy.

No sooner had this unwelcome penny dropped than, for the first time ever, a doctor made me a cup of coffee instead of the other way round. It was not the last time unexpected tables were turned in my military world. It was by no means always a rigid, unamusing one; the opposite was more often the case.

When hearing that I was to join the QA's, my ex-RAMC uncle said that as soon as I joined I would be sent on a course. He was right.

Edinburgh

After five months at Louise Margaret I drove up to Edinburgh to do a three month Special Care Baby Course at the famous Simpson Memorial Maternity Pavilion.

It was in a modern wing at the back of the (old) Edinburgh Royal Infirmary, with the Special Care unit on the top floor. The big windows had glorious views over The Meadows and away to the Pentland Hills, with the artificial ski slope on the latter a clear landmark.

The level of treatment and care was exemplary. The teaching was high powered but I managed to cope. One great memory is Christmas Day. Incubators not in use were stored in a large room with other equipment. On Christmas morning it was all pushed aside to enable a long table to be set up, and all the staff had breakfast together. The sister in charge apologised to the other QA and me, saying she realised Christmas in Scotland was not as much celebrated as in England. She then invited us to dinner in her home that evening. Her sister was a talented cook and we had a memorable meal, including our first ever taste of the classic Highland Atholl Brose, or rather, a close cousin which was even better. One of my best Christmases ever!

The atmosphere in the main hospital was almost palpable, so full of history was the building. Once I was sent into one of the corner towers to fetch some X-Rays and the atmosphere was memorable – hard to describe but perhaps a sense of the hundreds of people who had climbed those narrow stairs in the past. I have never forgotten the strange feeling.

A great bonus was having only a short walk to the Royal Mile and the old town, then down to Princes Gardens and the joys of the New Town. Explorations further afield were always interesting, including a day in St Andrews. My favourite small Scottish city, and we reached it by train. Sadly, that branch line was a Beeching victim, so long gone, but the excitement of crossing the Forth railway bridge is still part of any train journey going north from Edinburgh. Another, longer trip, took Margaret and I to Ellon, in Aberdeenshire, where in a small pub/hotel I slept under a duvet for the first time.

It was an incredible three months, despite a theft from my room, and two unpleasant experiences in very different circumstances. The day we went to a QA's funeral was a dreadful one. She was a nice girl I had known in LMMH and had died suddenly, cause unknown. The Brigadier had asked Margaret and I to represent her, but, against Regulations, I had not taken my No. Two suit to Edinburgh and had to wear civilian clothes. Far worse was to come.

The Major in charge of the Edinburgh MRS (Medical Reception Station, for sick soldiers) was tasked with organising transport. Her geography was non-existent, ditto any idea of driving times. The funeral was in the wilds of Perthshire and the weather forecast was poor. The army car was too small for four of us, and ordered too late to give enough time to get us there. We got lost.

It started to snow, quickly getting deeper; we had to find a farm, then drive through the farmyard to get to the church. We missed the service, arriving at the graveside in time to hear 'earth to earth, ashes to ashes'.

No wake, we had to leave to return the car on time, and I do not remember even speaking to anyone in the family. However the vicar accosted me and asked 'Did I not think that QAs were spoilt?' He persisted, while I was speechless at such insensitivity. To end this awful day, back in my room I discovered I had been burgled.

A twenty-first birthday present, a small luxan hide jewellery case was missing, one of a spate of thefts in the Nurses' Home. A few days later it was found, empty of course, thrown away in the main bus station. The main loss was the string of Ciro pearls, also a twenty-first birthday present, given to me by my parents because my mother treasured hers, and I had been glad to ask for a similar string.

There is a happy ending. The insurance money later enabled me to buy a string of cultured Mikimoto pearls, in Lane Crawford, the Harrods of Hong Kong.

The other unpleasant experience occurred in Anderson's, George Street; friends in Lochcarron had told me to go there when I wanted a kilt. It was an imposing store, large, historic, posh. Walls full of photographs of royalty, all wearing tartan of course.

That got me off on the wrong foot, no doubt. The rather snooty, elderly assistant informed me that ladies did not wear kilts, they wore kilt skirts. Next, I did not know what tartan I wanted. At the time I did not know of the family connections to the Douglases.

Having redeemed myself by choosing the Black Watch – by coincidence a military tartan therefore not associated with one clan or family, I was measured, name and address noted, and off I went to wait ten weeks until it would be ready for collection.

It was too tight. Madame gave me a talking to about the fit, reluctantly sent me away for three hours while it was to be 'eased'; and was even less happy on my return when once again it felt too tight. It was horrible standing up to her, but she agreed it must be altered. It would have to return to Glasgow and would not be ready until the New Year.

As the course ended in December I said it would have to be posted. I gave my address. Instead of Miss Sandilands, Nurses' Home Royal Infirmary, I became Captain Sandilands, QARANC Officers' Mess, Louise Margaret Maternity Hospital, Aldershot.

Never has anyone's attitude changed so abruptly. She was full of apologies – of course I was right, it would be dealt with as soon as possible ... Yuk.

When it arrived it was a perfect fit and I still have it. But it is too tight now...

Chapter 11

Hong Kong
1973–1975

FOLLOWING A FEW more months at LMMH, I was posted to Hong Kong.

'Trooping' was done by the RAF, and one afternoon I arrived at Brize Norton, where one found a normal airport style check-in desk. When my documents were checked there was obvious puzzlement; nothing was said but after a couple of minutes a senior man was called. He looked at the docs, looked at me, decided to spill the beans, laughed, and confided that I was listed as a male officer.

That sorted, no more problems. A comfortable flight, with a refuelling stop in the Seychelles, where we had to leave the aircraft, and wait in a garden area where many locals welcomed us, somewhat starved for varied entertainment it seemed. The heat was intense although it was the middle of the night; fruit drinks were available. In Hong Kong we landed at Kai Tak, the old civilian airport, the runway shared with the RAF, the far end stretching out into the harbour.

Some months later I watched a huge civilian aircraft skimming the tops of six storey blocks of flats in order to land safely. Standing in the road underneath with the undercarriage feeling only a few feet above my head was, shall I say, interesting.

Due to some hiccup no car arrived. The QAs who came to meet me commandeered a lift, which is how I came to arrive at the hospital in the back of a four ton truck – much to my father's amusement. The QA Mess was in a fifteen-storey tower block next to the hospital. My room was on the fourteenth floor, with a fantastic view over the harbour and across to Hong Kong Island, as well as looking down the Lai Mun Gap, through which all the biggest ships came, including a vast, ugly container ship, quite new in those days.

The big balcony was unusable. Noisy, as only Hong Kong could be, dusty, plagued with flying insects; a sad disappointment. In the corridor outside, usually down at the far end near the amah's work room, sat an enormous tarantula-type spider. Mercifully I never saw it moving.

The other local wildlife was a small green gecko which did move. One hot afternoon it appeared in my room and crawled along two walls, about waist height. Eventually I decided to treat it like a spider, so speaking most politely explained that although I knew it was harmless I really did not like it, so please would it leave my room. It sat and thought about it, then slowly turned, went back down to the bottom of the door, disappeared under the gap and never returned. (Later, in Nepal, I learned to live with all kinds of wildlife, including sharing a loo with six geckos. At least they stayed up near the ceiling.)

Hong Kong was wonderful. More than once I read, including in the *South China Morning Post*, that it was no place for middle-aged single women. Nonsense. The crowded, noisy cities of Kowloon on the mainland and Hong Kong Central on the Island; the boats in the typhoon harbours; ferries galore; the outer islands. Peaceful walking, fun orienteering, exploring islands – especially Cheung Chau at Festival time, the most traditional island. Remote areas of countryside, visiting villages and temples. Shopping!

The scores of nightclubs held no interest, except on one evening out with friends including men, I persuaded them to take us to one. We literally went down steps to the entrance, peered in and retreated. Saw little, but curiosity satisfied.

A friend of mine had nursed a helicopter pilot and subsequently he arranged for seven of us to have a trip in an RAF helicopter to a remote area of the New Territories, then to Lantau Island where we landed on a patch of English-like fine turf, on a col high up between the twin peaks of the island. He took us to see where our patients might come from, especially casualties from the training areas in the New Territories. Helicopters could land at the hospital, but at the last minute this was cancelled. We returned to Kai Tak instead, where the RAF had a small base in one corner of the airport. Then off to a party.

There is a monastery on Lantau Island and twice I stayed a night in the guesthouse. It was near a farm established to care for a herd of cows, which supplied fresh milk to the main hotels. Walking up the track from the monastery to the farm one passed the bull. He stood in a pen below the track, and it was quite something to look down on his huge back, but he disdained acknowledging passers by. The second time there I was on my own and a sweet young Chinese woman insisted on fetching and serving my food for me.

One of my favourite memories of my time in Hong Kong was an incident in the maternity unit one evening. I was working at the desk in the office of the lying-in ward, where we had shy and lovely 'Diddies', wives of the wonderful Gurkha soldiers.

An extremely smart Sergeant came in, crashed to attention on the other side of the desk, gave a terrific salute, and said 'Memsahib. My wife. She is wishing to be pissing.' (She had had a caesar.) Needless to say, he was not being rude, it is the recognised word the Gurkhas use. Nursing had long ago taught me to keep a straight face...

In the maternity unit we had three local Hong Kong girls, enrolled nurses, nice lasses. One of them got married and a couple of us were privileged to be invited to the traditional Chinese part of her three-day celebration. The first day had had a classic Christian white wedding, the second the Chinese ceremony Third day unknown, but a modern hooly with her friends hinted at. We sat at large round tables for ten. At each change of the many courses the table was cleared, including the white linen cloth, the wooden top folded in half and carried away. A new one, fully laid, replaced it. Slick and impressive.

Another, by all accounts very rare, privilege was to be taken by my amah, Chan, to her home on Hong Kong Island. A crowded, typical one room apartment in one of dozens of high rise blocks of flats, built to house the huge influx of Chinese refugees escaping Chairman Mao and his restrictions in the 1960s. Chan and her entire family – eight, I believe – lived in that space. A kitchen corner, bathroom corner, bunk beds, balcony covered with washing and plants; all cleverly arranged and neat.

Afterwards she insisted on taking me to Tiger Balm gardens, very famous and very popular with the Chinese. Hideous! Full of ghastly concrete, garishly coloured animals and other figures, on a steep hillside, exhausting to explore in the heat. Next she took me to an enormous, noisy, typical Dim Sum restaurant for lunch – the Chinese take all their pleasures with as much noise as possible! A fascinating, unforgettable day.

Chapter 12

Nepal
1974–1975

POSTINGS TO NEPAL were for nine months, preferably always from Hong Kong. As I was keen to go to Nepal, I was urged to see Matron as soon as possible, despite only having just arrived; my request was greeted with pleasure, so after six months off I went. The week before leaving, I spent at Stanley Bay on the far side of Hong Kong Island, learning to sail a dinghy.

At my farewell interview with the Commanding Officer, he remarked that he could not think of a more useless course to do before being posted to the Himalayas

We flew in an RAF plane, landing in a far corner of Calcutta airport for refuelling. Despite a delay we were not allowed off the plane, the implication was that we were not welcome in India.

Dharan is 140 miles east of Kathmandu, and after landing some of us transferred to a local airline which flew us to Biratnagar, on flat land near the Indian border. From there a car drove us north through a band of open jungle between the Indian Border and the first foothills of the Himalayas. Dharan is a small town at the bottom of them – a busy area hub, especially as a major track up into the mountains starts just beyond it. Although a thousand feet above sea level the land slopes so gently it felt flat, and most of it was open forest called the Terai, where tigers used to roam.

Almost within yards beyond the town, to the north, the first true edge of the mountains looked formidable. Walls stretched as far as one could see, both horizontally and vertically. In fact not quite as vertical as they appeared, for at the foot began the track up to the first ridge,

3000ft above. Porters scurried up and down, with mind-blowing loads on their backs, mainly in huge woven 'dhokas', the Nepalese version of backpacks but always with a band round the forehead. Occasionally, instead of a dhoka they carried several sheets of corrugated iron or other unwieldy loads. They tended to move almost at a run, while bent double under their burdens.

I arrived in May, and in June went up to the chalet, built on the top of the first ridge, a gift from Lord Nuffield. Famous for the loo with a view of distant Kanchenjunga. It was a stiff two hour climb, with frequent pauses to allow descending porters to pass, and once, even a donkey. Another surprise was an old lady in a basket chair perched on a man's back. There was no other way of accessing the area in our part of Nepal.

At the top of the ridge we left the busy 'main road', turning right to make our way to the chalet, another 1,000ft up. Matron nearly did not come, as she had been several times, but she was a keen walker and sad that she was about to be posted home. The monsoon was due to break and I was assured that there would be no view of Everest.

Not only was it visible, I was the first to see it, which was pretty ridiculous. Outside my room in the Mess was an outline diagram of all the main peaks, with each one named. Liking maps I had studied it with interest. Not long after the beginning of our almost vertical walk to the chalet, a much quieter track allowed time to look around,

Looking across ridge after ridge of hills, and past the 'free-standing' and particularly attractive Makalu, I was remarkably confident that I had identified Everest. At first no one would believe me but then everyone agreed and Matron was absolutely delighted. She had never seen it during any of her previous treks.

Too bad she left. Her replacement detested outdoor life, and most reluctantly gave me permission to go trekking, daring me to return ill. Happily when I returned I was probably the fittest I have ever been in my life.

Warned before leaving Hong Kong that there would only be one week of leave during our nine months (normal tour length) and not even that if some emergency occurred, the policy changed soon after my arrival. Matron sent for me one day and asked when I would like a week off. In addition sisters were not supposed to do night duty, but I 'specialled' a very ill woman for a week and was then astonished to be given a week of nights off.

Days off for two weeks could sometimes be put together making a long weekend. The result of all this was not only a week-long trek with a doctor's wife and four porters, but also a week in Kashmir; three nights in Pokhara (west Nepal); a long weekend in Darjeeling; one in Delhi and Agra, and at least one in Kathmandu. It was in a back street of Kathmandu, at 10 pm one night, I bought my typical local drum

For many years Kathmandu had my record for more take-offs and landings than any other airport. It included a one hour, very early morning flight which gained me a certificate confirming that this morning I had 'Greeted Sargamatha', the Nepali name for Everest.

Flying from Biratnagar to Kathmandu meant always flying west with views of the highest mountain peaks all the way – sometimes hazy but rarely lost in cloud. Best of all was the flight in a little six-seater aeroplane, which took off from our golf course. I was put in the front seat, and of course small planes fly low and slow, so all the way the views were exceptional.

There was a huge amount to do in Dharan, and though I played, and enjoyed, croquet a couple of times, I never got around to trying golf. Dinner parties were frequent, thanks to all the married families in the Cantonment, but three of my main memories concerned Mess life.

On my first evening, a schoolteacher came in swinging a racket. Without a trace of irony she said 'Anyone for tennis?' It set the tone, and in my first letter home I wrote that the Cantonment had passed the First World War but did not appear to have to have reached the Second. That was in the QA Mess, but two more tales were both in the RAMC Mess.

On Sunday evenings we had a film, projected on to a screen in the garden of the Mess, with the audience sitting along the veranda. Ladies were allowed to enter through the bar, but under no circumstances via the ante-room (sitting room) next door. Totally, always, out-of-bounds to all women. As for the dining room, heaven forbid! For pure badness, once I put a whole foot over the threshold of the ante-room – but not when any men were looking.

Much later, not long before returning to Hong Kong, major work in the QA Mess kitchen closed our dining room for several weeks. We even had to have breakfast in the RAMC Mess. On my first morning there I had a particularly interesting conversation with one of the most confirmed old diehards in the cantonment – he survived, and so did the Mess.

On Christmas Day I was warned to listen to the Cantonment radio at 11 am. Greetings to me were broadcast by my mother, then my sister asked me to be Godmother to my nephew, born in August. It transpired the Admin Officer had written to all the families asking if they would like to record a taped message to be played on Christmas Day.

When back home I heard all about making the tape, and I told about my phone call from Delhi – a complicated tale.

The family knew nothing about recording, so phoned BBC Radio Oxford for help. They were invited there to record and all went well, except that they wanted my nephew Julian to gurgle or make a noise, to 'introduce' him to his potential Godmother. Unfortunately this 4-month-old baby did not cooperate. He was rolled on a table, nearly thrown on the floor, but refused to wake up. Afterwards the family went home with my parents for the evening, and so were there when I rang home out of the blue.

En route back from my week in Kashmir, I was staying overnight in the YMCA hostel in Delhi having been told it was very good, and also that ladies were allowed to stay. Indeed, there was even a telephone in my room. In Kashmir a man had wanted to draw my astrological chart, but needed a fairly exact time of birth, which I did not know. So now was a chance to find out. Reception assured me a normal three-hour wait for a connection would only be half an hour tonight.

Up in my room organisation was needed. The phone had a short cord, only reaching from the far wall to the foot of the bed, so I put it there, with a list beside it of things to remember to say. More than an hour later, with reluctance, I cancelled the call and went to bed, as I had to be up at 4 am to catch the Kathmandu flight (the one when I sat watching the Himalayas with a G&T in my hand – at 8 o'clock in the morning...)

At 2.30 am came the message 'This is your call', and I exclaimed 'Oh, I'm not ready!' Bedside light hard to reach, ditto phone, no list to hand – and my mother saying she was not pleased that I was not ready to speak to her. No time to explain, but the extraordinary thing was hearing Julian, awake and making baby noises. Which is how I met my nephew for the first time – in India.

The other Christmas Day memory, often quoted, was a drive, a first in a Range Rover. It was the most treasured possession of a retired diplomat, and despite 20,000 miles on Nepal's awful roads and tracks, in dust, mud and rain if allowed out during a monsoon, it was pristine outside and in, with immaculate, beautiful cream leather upholstery, maintained lovingly by the Nepalese driver.

The diplomat was visiting friends in the Cantonment for Christmas, but wanted to visit a water tap near the foot of the path up to Dhankuta, the one just beyond Dharan. He had organised the installation of many taps, and was keen to see how this one was faring. Three of us were invited to join him for the drive, which included navigating across a wide stony, dried-up riverbed. Magic. Blissfully comfortable. I have coveted a Range Rover ever since. Also coveted a kukri, and was able to have one made for me. A proper one, with a lethal blade, but in a silver scabbard intricately chased. The design includes a minute gold QA badge, and a pretty butterfly – symbol for a woman. It is beautiful, and very precious.

One of the joys of Dharan was being in the west of Nepal, so not spoilt by the hippy trails to Kathmandu. In Pokhara the children always ran up, hands outstretched, begging persistently for 'one rupee'. In Dharan we were happy they had not learnt that ploy.

Hippy trails or not, a few years ago Nepal was voted by a travel company as the most beautiful in the world. In 2017/18 either *Lonely Planet* – or *Rough Guide* said Scotland was the most beautiful. Scotland wins because it has more variety, and it has the sea. But never doubt, Nepal is second. (Incidentally, Gurkha soldiers have an affinity with Scotland, not least as they enjoy the bagpipes, and have their own Regimental pipers. When in the UK, visiting Scotland is always a goal for them.)

When it was time to fly back to Hong Kong the baggage allowance was one hundred pounds, Main baggage separate, via the infamous MFO boxes – Military Forwarding Office. There were few people about, and little action at check-in, so I heaved my suitcase on to the floor scales; surprised and delighted to see it weighed spot on one hundred pounds. Then someone turned up and laughed at me, saying there was no problem. When we boarded all became clear. The fuselage of the Britannia looked huge, because it was almost empty. My case was in a small row of bags strapped down together and looking almost silly, lost in the vast space. No wonder I was laughed at.

At the far end two rows of seats sat in one half of the plane, facing backwards as all passenger seats do in the RAF – 'The safest airline in the world'. Anne, the other QA returning to Hong Kong, and two RAF ground crew, were the only other passengers. We could choose our seats, were plied with endless offers of fruit juice and coffee, asked what time we would like our main meal, and invited to go up to the cockpit at any time. To this day I regret not going as soon as we received the invitation, because I missed flying over Rangoon, so did not see the many temples, which would have been wonderful.

Most memorable was the crew playing cricket. Great use of the empty space! The ball was rolled up newspaper, the bats forgotten – maybe rolled up paper too.

We were invited to the cockpit for the landing at Kai Tak; unforgettable as we skimmed over the blocks of flats and then taxied towards a dip in the harbour…. Of course that unique flight is an exceptional memory, but there is an astonishing postscript.

For many years while working in Oxford, my sister had a friend, Sue, whose husband had been in the RAF. They retired, moved to Suffolk, and Richard wrote a book about his life, and time in the RAF as an Air Loadmaster. In 2019, after one of her holidays with them, Jenny borrowed the book for me to read. Richard reminisced about flying in the Far East, flying in a Britannia from Kathmandu to Hong Kong, playing cricket in the empty fuselage. Jenny contacted Sue, she told Richard – he checked his log book, I had checked my diary. Same date. Apparently the only day ever that cricket was played; a total one off.

It was probably Richard who laughed at me when I was so chuffed about my case weighing the exact limit.

The final six months back in Hong Kong were uneventful. It was disappointing to learn that the orienteering I'd previously enjoyed had become much more serious and competitive, so it sounded as if the fun had gone out of it – but irrelevant for me in any case as there was no longer a place in the team, having been away for so long.

One day I went out to the New Territories, to visit a Gurkha Welfare Officer who had been a friend in Nepal and was now based in the Gurkha Training Centre in a remote area.

She took me for a walk into the firing ranges, along a track with bushes on either side alive with myriads of butterflies, all sizes and colours. Fabulous, and a reminder that Army training areas are frequently havens of life for both plants and animals, peaceful when no humans are making a racket, and where civilians are rarely allowed to roam, so everything wild thrives. In England, Lulworth is an example.

Chapter 13

Tidworth

1975–1978

WHEN DUE HOME after two years in Hong Kong we were allowed to choose our next posting. Subject to ... all the usual caveats.

My request for Tidworth was granted. Chosen for two reasons: not too far from home, and also where my father had lived as a little boy, 1907–1910. The house is still there, the current tenant was a doctor who promised to show me round inside one day but unfortunately never did. It was a tall, three storey house – from the nursery on the top floor my father had fallen out of the window. Lucky not to be killed, he had a scar on the side of his head for the rest of his life.

Not being too far from home was important. While in Nepal an enigmatic letter from my father arrived, merely referring to my mother's chemotherapy. I rushed off to my doctor friend, Helen, hoping against hope that chemo might be for something other than cancer. No. Later it transpired that a twenty-page letter from my mother, with the whole story, never reached Nepal. Fortunately, by the time I returned she had recovered and life at home was normal.

By 1975 obstetricians were trying to control deliveries. In Oxford, at booking clinics, patients would be given a date for induction! The idea was to have virtually all deliveries between Mondays to Fridays, during normal working hours, when all the main ancillary staff would be on duty if help was needed. Mercifully our two obstetricians in Tidworth did not agree with 'Meddlesome Midwifery' so the unit was straightforward. So straightforward I remember few details.

The senior Consultant, Colonel Peake, was an old-fashioned gentleman, soon to retire. He used to invite newly posted-in midwives to dinner at his home. I had a lovely evening there, and learnt that he and his wife were close friends of Mr Dumoulin and his wife; Mr Dumoulin was a quiet, excellent obstetrician in Plymouth. My favourite consultant.

A story in Plymouth told of two schoolgirls on a bus, when one is overheard telling the other that her mother is expecting a baby. The friend refuses to believe it, 'Yes it is true. You ask your father'! Apocryphal? Mr Dumoulin was her father.

Colonel Peake's permanent home was in Berkshire, and he was said to do farming as a profession and obstetrics as a hobby. He told me a tale himself which made my hair stand on end. He and his wife had a brand new car, his wife was especially delighted with it. A week after getting it a friend offered him a load of special, fresh, smelly manure – so Colonel Peake shovelled it into the boot just as it was, straight on to the new carpet lining, not in a container, nothing underneath, no sacks, tarpaulin or waterproof sheet, nothing. He was very happy. His wife was not. But what a lovely man he was.

One glorious memory is being on night duty in the summer and listening to the larks, keeping an ear open for the earliest. 2.55 am. There were many on Salisbury Plain, always a great joy.

One day my friends Margaret and Christopher came for the day. Margaret and I had been friends since starting our training together at the Wingfield when we were 17 years old. Now all three of us had our fortieth birthdays. An amusing thought, for me, if I'd even thought of it at all, so it was a shock to discover that both of them considered it absolutely dreadful. We had wandered over to some event on the polo field, where I could not resist the lure of an ice cream van and bought three of the biggest cornets, which had to be eaten in public of course. An absolute No-No in our schooldays. Too old? Life over? Rubbish!

On another day, my cousin Ann with her husband Rex came up from Somerset with their children Mary and Claire. We took a picnic up into the woods beyond the shops on the Ludgershall road, where suddenly we saw a white rabbit, and quickly realised it was a domestic one. Far too vulnerable to be loose up there, but no houses nearby, so I captured it.

On the way back to the Mess we stopped at the police station and sent Ann – daughter of a policeman – to report our find. Her reception? Dogs, yes. Rabbits, no. End of conversation. Her father no help, an irrelevance and never mentioned.

In my room – at the time in Tidworth House (when no longer the QARANC Mess it reverted to its original name of Tedworth House) there was a tall wicker laundry basket. Rex disagreed with rabbits etc., being kept as pets, but in the circumstances took the rabbit back to Yeovil in the laundry basket. He was named Portland L. Tidworth (why Portland L?) and lived far beyond the normal allotted span of rabbits.

Chapter 14

Personnel Selection Officer

QATC 1977–1980

FROM TIDWORTH I DID the Junior Officers' Course at the QA Training Centre. A talk on Personnel Selection was interesting, and I said so. Before long I was PSO. My three years in Aldershot, as Personnel Selection Officer, were some of the most enjoyable of my career.

For the QA's girls needed to be right for nursing, but also for army life. Potential student nurses, for State Registration training, with five 'O' levels or more, were selected by a different system, including interviews by Sister Tutors.

All the others came via Personnel Selection; State Enrolled training to become practical assistant nurses; Ward Stewardesses; Dental Clerk Assistants and Clerical Assistants. The applicants had already been through a Recruiting Office selection. Those considered suitable were sent to the Training Centre for two nights, living with the recruits, watching a film on life in the Corps and the careers available, and given talks by a Sergeant. Finally they had an individual interview with a PSO, and were given an acceptance or rejection verdict before leaving.

My PS boss was a WRAC officer, an anomaly which stemmed from Selection being a 'Big Army' group, and QARANC the newest branch. Major Margaret Athoe and I got on well together but first there were introductory courses to be done. A week at PS HQ in Sutton Coldfield followed by a week in Beaconsfield at an RAEC Army School of Education. Royal Army Educational Corps; NEVER to be called Royal Army Education Corps.

Sutton Coldfield is a bit of a blur, though as a group we gelled quickly. Beaconsfield, by contrast, is remembered all too clearly, mainly for negative reasons.

It was a huge establishment and the Officers' Mess was boasted as having the tallest brick building in the country. My room was on the ninth floor of fifteen storeys. Dirty, boiling hot, the window opened no more than three inches, no staff on duty as it was a Sunday evening. Hence no clean sheets to replace the disgusting ones used by the previous occupant – not just a lone inhabitant of this single room... My complaint to the cleaning lady next morning was met with indifference. Oddly, not long afterwards a very senior officer was telling of a similar discovery on arrival in a new Mess. Unlike my Keep Quiet and Carry On effort, he told of causing uproar, calling out the Duty Officer and goodness knows who else to deal with the situation.

Venturing down for breakfast I made a boob trying to find the form in the vast dining room, but the stewardesses were unhelpful. The ante room (sitting room) was equally vast, with a subdued, formal atmosphere, not at all relaxing, though perhaps not surprising given the extraordinary mix of students. A Brigadier learning Arabic, Arabs learning English, Israelis learning English, civilian diplomats and service personnel learning Russian, and elsewhere senior Other Ranks attending numerous courses of varying length and complexity.

The rest of my group were housed in the Annexe so I always had to go to the Mess alone, grateful to see a familiar face sometimes. One abiding memory is the craft room. We were taken there one day, to produce a simple poster. It was a big room packed with first class equipment for every kind of art and craft imaginable, paradise for practical folk but sadly not for me. Margaret Athoe came to visit our course and my fellow members liked her, which was a cheering moment in a dreary week. One of our tasks was to give a practical demonstration of some aspect of our normal work, but even that gave me a headache. Intending to show how to bath a baby our instructor protested for some forgotten reason, but swapping to giving an injection provoked another unfriendly reaction. I was rejected on going to the Medical Centre to beg for a syringe, being advised in no uncertain terms that the Medical Centre did not provide any equipment to any student. Beaconsfield was not a happy place.

Once installed in my own department at the QA Training Centre, Margaret Athoe was seldom met, but one day she invited three of us to a dinner at the WRAC HQ Mess in Guildford, and on one happy occasion she took me as her guest to the Royal Academy Summer Exhibition, a huge treat.

We also enjoyed each others' company driving to Woolwich for the annual conference of Recruiting Officers and Selection Personnel. It was fun telling her about one of my favourite books, *We Joined the Navy*, mentioned ages ago. It begins with an Admiralty Interview Board and is hilarious from page one, though with occasional serious insights. A question asked of every candidate was what did they notice about a picture on the wall, an unremarkable watercolour of a boat in a harbour. One dimwit was hard put to it to describe the boat as a yacht. Another candidate described the boat, the state of the tide, and possible location of the harbour, but the best answer of all I quote here in full:

> It's a picture of a ketch, coming out on the evening ebb tide. Two men on deck, which means two girls below cooking supper. The harbour is on the South coast, probably by the shape of the hills and the red soil, Devon or possibly Dorset. Racing pennant, dinghy lashed on deck, spinnaker boom lying up for'd, they've probably just finished a day's racing and are on their way home to the next place round the point before closing time. They're just passing a starboard hand buoy with what looks like a wreck buoy close inshore. Leading mark on the hill.

Although I didn't give Margaret quite all this detail, she loved the gist of it, though do not think there was ever any thought of using a picture question in our own selection procedures. What I do remember is that it helped to pass the time on a long and tedious section of the South Circular road.

For about 300 years Woolwich was home to the Royal Artillery. The main building was famous for having the longest classical facade in the country, but by the 1970s much behind it had been demolished or modernised, though not the grand entrance hall or breathtaking dining hall. Eating my breakfast under a couple of tons of a chandelier was an experience to be savoured. There were three other identical ones too, the four unforgettable, enormous and stunning. Also unforgettable, enormous and stunning was the Gunners' collection of silver, such a big horde it was housed in a purpose-built room at one side of the main entrance hall, full of floor to ceiling glass display cases.

On my first visit we were just given a buffet supper but a subsequent one gave me two more never-to-be-forgotten memories. We were treated to a full-blown formal dinner, seated at two immensely long and impeccably laid tables. Before the port and Loyal Toast the tables were cleared, leaving only the single full-length white tablecloth in place. At either end a steward stationed himself, and an air of expectancy descended – anticipating what?

A gentle drum roll began, the stewards began to twist the cloth, faster and faster as the drum rolled to a crescendo, then Wham! the cloth was released. From the top it snaked at tremendous speed down the middle of the table to be gathered up at the bottom, about 30ft away. A brilliant performance, followed by the best port I have ever tasted, a 19-year-old vintage. A magnificent and privileged evening indeed.

Back down to earth in QATC, someone once shook her head at me, complaining about girls I had approved. For once in my life I had a prompt answer. 'You should have seen the ones I kept out!'

Our small department was originally a bit hugger-mugger in the main building, but then we moved moved to ideal rooms in the old stable block just inside the main gate. My office was in what had been the kitchen; my deputy, a Captain, next door. Down a short passage a Sergeant and Clerk did admin in a third office, then a large room for talks and films. Four applicants I remember in particular.

A pleasant, very suitable girl, was keen to work in operating theatres. As an Enrolled nurse that was not an option – ditto a good many other specialities. However, this lass had four 'O' Levels, so I encouraged her to go away, gain her fifth 'O' Level, train in a civilian hospital, and return to us to join as an officer. Several years later I was stopped in a corridor by a QA officer I did not recognise. She thanked me most gratefully for my advice – and she was working in theatre.

Another girl, big-bosomed and nearly bursting out of a khaki safari-style shirt, was an army daughter. It was almost comical, with hindsight, seeing her determination to join, with the all too obvious intention of reorganising whatever and whoever she considered necessary. She was not given the chance.

Another very nice girl wanted to be a nurse, but not in the QAs. She was not from a service background, but her parents thought she would be in a safe, controlled environment. She had a boyfriend, knew which civilian hospital she wanted to train in, and I sent her away with best wishes for doing just that. Mentally giving two fingers to her over-protective, dictatorial parents and wondering how she would fare when she told them.

The fourth girl was the most memorable of all. She was from 'Camp' , the wild open country in the Falkland Islands. As it happened, shortly before she arrived an interesting article about 'Camp' had been published in the *Telegraph* weekend magazine so I was able to discuss life there with her. She was tall, with an unusual Christian name. Intelligent, and with four 'O' Levels, she was sent away to get her fifth and train as a State Registered nurse.

When visiting the Falklands thirty years later, from several options I chose a visit to Long Island Farm in order to see 'Camp'. The bus drove for an hour on farm property before reaching the farmstead, where we were entertained with tea and shown various interesting aspects of farm life. 'That's my cousin! Una!' exclaimed the farmer's wife when I mentioned a tall girl with an unusual name.

They had been close when young, Una spending a lot of time on the farm. There was a slight hint of her not being very happy at home, but also she had always been ambitious, hence her travel to England. She did get her fifth 'O' Level, did train in a civilian hospital, did join the QAs, and spent several years in the Corps. Now, in 2008, came astonishing news. She was teaching critical care in two universities; the West of England and A N Other. Married, living in Bristol, six months ago had triplets and also had a 2-year-old son! She'd had to be 17 to be eligible for Selection, so now was certainly a mature Mum in her forties. An amazing story. Her cousin Glenda Watson promised to pass on my greetings.

Going home was the sad aspect of life during Personnel Selection. My mother was frequently not very well and at one point was admitted to the Churchill Hospital, where she was found to be seriously anaemic, mercifully easily treatable and not a return of her cancer. So, huge relief – but not for long

In December 1978 (the only year I never kept a diary – odd) after a very difficult week I went home on the Friday. Three days in Harrogate on a useless course on interview techniques had been followed by a brief but unusual stay in the Lake District with 'Aunty Simpo', my mother's oldest friend. Many wonderful holidays with her now left me with a reminder that when a neighbour during my pre-3-year-old days, she could be a real disciplinarian.

My bed in Harrogate was so uncomfortable I had had very little sleep, and arrived very tired after driving across the Pennines. Aunty scolded, saying she did not know what to do with me, but all I wanted was to go to bed. I thought it a bad end to a bad week, but worse was to come.

Back at home, the doctor had been, and they had agreed it was time for my mother to go into Sir Michael Sobel House. It was only the second hospice in the UK, a completely new concept to all except Dr Cicely Saunders and a few others. Many people deplored the idea of terminal care away from home, but my mother embraced it at once, even before she had cancer, and I agreed with her.

An ambulance had been arranged to collect her on the following Monday. I feared an extremely difficult weekend, especially as she would be tired after a visit from her sister and family, but perhaps she felt that the end of her struggle was in sight.

Whatever the reason she was in great form all the time, very happy, so it a was wonderful couple of days. On a gloriously sunny Monday morning my father and I sat in the bedroom with her until the ambulance arrived, around lunch time on 11 December.

We saw her settled into a ward with half a dozen patients and with her bed by a window. Mondays were encouraged as no visiting days, to give both patients and families respite. No visiting rules were absolute and we could have stayed but were happy to follow advice. We left, but as we walked out I looked at the other patients and thought Mummy had at least three months to go. This despite her conviction, since before last Christmas, that she would die before this one.

She died the next day. Peacefully, after telling Sister how much she had enjoyed her lunch.

Poor Jenny had an appalling time. With 4-year-old Julian and 2-year-old Alison, she had gone to lunch with 'Brumpy', our father, before going to the Hospice, but as they were at the front door with their coats on the phone rang with the news. Jenny had bought a tiny jigsaw for the children to play with on a bed table during their visit; she later said that, back in the house, she had never done a jigsaw so frantically.

I had gone back to work, but was sent on compassionate leave as soon as I told the Commandant about Jenny's call. She said I should not return until after Christmas, so that gave me three weeks at home. When back in the Mess, seeing another member whom I did not know very well, I told her my news. 'Oh, these things happen' said she, and waltzed away. Hmmm.

My great regret was that my mother died alone. Very early in my days at King's I discovered that deaths did not upset me. I mean the actual event. Even if a patient was unconscious I wanted someone to be with them, to hold their hand and say goodbye, so it saddened me that my mother had no one.

Nine weeks after my mother died so did Maureen, in February 1980. She was a special friend, my first flatmate in Plymouth. Like my other three flatmates she married a Naval officer from Manadon, but he had retired and was at a Theological College near Nottingham when this awful tragedy struck. Maureen had worked in the Special Care Baby Unit, loved babies and longed for her own, so a six-year-wait after her wedding seemed endless. Then good news, as three babies gradually arrived. But that meant she died leaving a 7-year-old, a 3-year-old and a 1-year-old toddler. Unable to go to her funeral, in freezing weather I went next door to the Garrison Church and sat quietly remembering her and thinking of the family she had left.

Personnel Selection was a Monday to Friday timetable, so with every weekend free I was able to go home, to help my sister to look after my father – an undomesticated gentleman. He did try hard to look after himself, but was not equipped with housekeeping skills. He was under strict instructions never to touch the new washing machine. Neither Jenny nor I trusted him with anything mechanical; his record with anything other than cars was dire.

One day he astonished me by saying he had always wanted to go to America. He'd never mentioned it before, and I would have guessed it to be the last place he would want to go. A cheering aspect of his life was now having a drug which stopped his Parkinson-like tremor. For years he refused to eat or drink in public, not even with family, but spilling his tea was no longer a fear so a trip seemed a bit of a fillip for him. So we went – but our adventures are a story for another time.

Chapter 15

Princess Alexandra's RAF Hospital Wroughton
1980–1982

AFTER THREE YEARS as PSO, and being promoted to Major, I was posted to Princess Alexandra's Royal Air Force Hospital, Wroughton, in a beautiful area half way up the Marlborough Downs above Swindon. It was a thoughtful posting as it meant I could still get home to Oxford easily to help look after my father.

PAH had been amalgamated with Tidworth, so now had RAMC and QA staff too. Initially the amalgamation went very badly as the RAF Commanding officer was so unwelcoming, even being rude to incoming senior RAMC Consultants.

If PSO had not unexpectedly intervened I would have been one of the first QAs there, but by the time I arrived three years later a new CO was excellent, and everyone had settled down. The QA's, not really surprisingly, were desperately short of sisters with paediatric qualifications. With my Special Care Baby Certificate I was put in charge of the Children's Ward, luckily not a busy one as facilities were limited. Seriously ill children were sent to the new Radcliffe Infirmary in Oxford, which I was lucky enough to experience when taking a very sick baby there; a fantastic unit with a wonderful Sister in charge.

In order to improve morale, and cooperation between the Army and the RAF, the new CO had inaugurated the Halton to Wroughton Walk. It was designated an official Exercise, in order that transport and other back-up details could be used, and was called 'Petit Mash', after the daft TV comedy series set in a United States field hospital in Korea.

122

Our Petit Mash was soon better known as the Wiltshire Walkabout. Informal, and for all ranks, it was a two day, sixty mile trek along the Icknield Way in the Chiltern Hills to the River Thames, then along the Berkshire Downs Ridgeway to Wroughton. We had to be in teams of three and spend the first night under canvas on the edge of the playing fields near RAF Halton hospital, before walking thirty miles to the river. The CO ferried everyone across the Thames in his Gemini rubber dinghy to the Beetle and Wedge in Moulsford. (Venue of my wedding reception thirteen years later.) Not for liquid refreshment, but for transport to a camp that was ready for us, tucked away in a fold of the Downs. My team leader, Helen, had arranged for her brother to bring a caravan, so we slept in luxury that night. Incidentally the Officers' Mess at Halton was in one of Rothschild's mansions but sadly we never saw it, much less set foot inside.

Carma was the third member of Helen's team, a lovely PM (Princess Mary's RAF Nursing Service) who was blighted by being over 6ft tall. Everyone was delighted for her when, a few years later, she acquired a boyfriend said to be even taller than her. Sadly, he ditched her – at least so I heard. As so often in the Forces, news, and rumours, travelled, but with no confirmation.

For the second day we woke once again to perfect walking weather. Dry and sunny but not too hot, May at its best. This was the third Walkabout, one had been very cold and one had had pouring rain, so we were most blessed. It was also the last one, for reasons unknown. I had done four long practice walks, but the final two/three miles were a real slog, largely because my feet were covered in blisters, because despite several efforts I had not been able to find any pure wool socks, and the ones with some nylon content were as unsatisfactory as feared. However, not only did the three of us make it, we won the Women's trophy!

Several days later, at a presentation ceremony, the CO took me to look at a table covered in a variety of figurines. Not knowing if I was supposed to admire them, I muttered some non-committal remark – though I suspect he would not have minded, indeed probably agreed, had I given my honest opinion. They were ghastly. Cheap, ugly, overblown, badly designed; ornate columns topped by triumphant gilt figurines, arms aloft.

Helen, Carma and I each received one of them, with a winged, torch-bearing female on top and a small plate at the base inscribed

'No 1 Ladies'. Then I was presented with a second one; this time with a trunks-wearing, laurel-wreath-waving bloke. Given to me with apologies, because no one had imagined a woman over forty qualifying, the plate bore the legend 'Veteran'.

It was odd enough, after Basic Fitness Training was introduced, to find myself running round an international standard Tartan track in Aldershot, but for a determined non-athlete these hideous trophies are actually treasured, and now sit on top of a cabinet in my bathroom.

TA Exercise

The blisters on my feet had all the skin trimmed off them in A&E – the worst possible treatment, not some wonderful new one as I imagined. Within days, while still hobbling, I was sent on my first ever genuine Army Exercise. As an Umpire. Ridiculous really. I had never set eyes on an exercise, let alone been a player, so I hadn't a clue what to expect.

It happened because Big Guns had decided that the TA – Territorial Army – sometimes called Weekend Soldiers, should be integrated much more closely with the Regular army. The TAs were civilians who met once a week in drill halls, did an occasional weekend exercise, and a week long one once a year. Fairly or unfairly, often considered as social clubs. All a far cry from Reservists in the twenty-first century, who play their part brilliantly in every conflict in which the UK gets involved.

So, off I go, complete with combat kit and army boots, to HQ Southern Command at Wilton, near Salisbury. The senior QA, was very friendly. I was to be on duty at night, welcome to have dinner in the Mess beforehand if I would like to, then willing to drive myself out to Westdown Camp about fifteen miles away. Hence I discovered I could drive in army boots, but having first had a delicious dinner which included my first ever avocado mousse. Doubtless HQ had Class One chefs, not just to indulge senior officers there, but for entertaining visiting VIPs both civilian and military.

It was always said that after the Second World War army catering improved more than any other branch. Certainly by the late 1970s army chefs were banned from civilian cooking competitions because they kept winning everything.

Invitations to meals at Catering Corps HQ in Aldershot were highly prized – too bad one never came my way. Incidentally, QA and RAMC Messes always had Class One chefs. They were needed in hospitals due to the need for their knowledge of special diets, but they hated this work. So, a normal two-year posting would be for one year in the hospital kitchen, with the other in one of the Officers' Messes – greatly to our good fortune.

At Westdown both my Colonel and the Senior Umpire told me to take it easy, as I was still hobbling quite badly. On arrival I was told to put my feet up, on a sofa in an office, where I stayed until the early hours of the next morning. Not a common way of being on Exercise – but a godsend as it turned out, because I spent the time reading from A to Z a manual on Operating Orders. Interesting, helpful and an invaluable aid to this rooky umpire.

My chief memory has nothing to do with the actual exercise. An army doctor at Wroughton had lent me his woolly-pulley, but he had done a parachute course and so had Para wings on the sleeve. It was astonishing how many soldiers noticed them, often with surprise, and congratulated me, so frequent, apologetic explanations were necessary.

At the end of the exercise Colonel Chamberlain asked me to write a report which was a nasty shock. However I managed a page or so, and never heard any more about it.

An irrelevant but pleasant memory ended this rather odd experience. Peggy McGilp was the daytime QA Umpire, and before going our separate ways we went to visit the Wilton carpet factory shop. With no intention or expectation of buying anything, I fell for a Chinese rug, hanging on a wall in the midst of a sea of plain colours. Having bought one in Hong Kong I knew enough to recognise something of the quality of this one, and the reasonable price. The colours were pale, unusual but attractive. Why it was there seemed strange, but no matter. Peggy kindly bought it for me – or rather paid, as I had left my cheque book at Wroughton. We remained friends until her death.

Back at Wroughton, as Christmas approached on the Children's ward the popular TV programme for children, *Blue Peter*, announced the object for its annual charity collection. Used stamps. Previous things had been old keys, tinfoil, etc. I suggested the staff might like to make a collection. It took off. We even had a big boxful delivered from Matron at RAF Hospital Wegberg, in Germany.

The result was an invitation to take three nurses to BBC TV Centre in Shepherd's Bush, to watch a *Blue Peter* programme being made.

There were some mutterings because one of the girls I chose to take was a scruffy lass with a dubious record of poor behaviour. Later on I heard that her equally scruffy husband had dismantled his motorbike – on the kitchen table… And later still that she was court martialled, though I've no idea why.

However, she had thrown her heart and soul into collecting stamps, getting more than anyone else. I had reason to believe she had rarely had any praise or reward in her life, so I was actually pleased to include her in the expedition. I think she could hardly believe it, but despite the special occasion it did not help her preparations. When the rest of us arrived at her married quarter to collect her I was stunned by the state of her shoes We were wearing our uniforms, which usually meant shoes so highly polished you could nearly see your face in them. Hers looked as if they had neither polish nor a brush since the day they were issued. She was sent back indoors to clean them, but they were little better when she returned. Probably no polish in the house? There was no time to pursue it.

I drove us to Television Centre, where we received a friendly welcome, were told where to park the car, then go into Reception. One member of staff took one look at us in our uniforms and said 'Oh, do let me look at your shoes'. Her reason why has been forgotten; just the utter disbelief at the request, not to mention acute embarrassment.

After the show we were taken to meet the famous editor, Biddy Baxter. She was pleasant, yes, but there was something formidable about her; she had not achieved so much without a steely side. Did she notice the shoes…?

Around the time of our BBC adventure a topic which hit the headlines was the possibility of male midwives. A handful of men wanted to qualify, and provoked fierce debate. One day several young nurses were in the office and arguments began. Mostly anti-males.

When I thought they had gone on long enough I just asked how they would feel if, when in labour, in pain, wanting help, Greg walked in. Instant end of arguments.

Greg was a small, kind, happily married man with two nice children, a boy and girl aged 6 and 8. No contest, Greg would be more than welcome in a labour ward. To all of us he was a superb practical nurse, loved by everyone, staff, parents, and children. Even had he wanted to, he could not train as a midwife because he was only an Enrolled Nurse. Matron had tasked me with trying to persuade him to do his Registered Nurse training, but he refused. Probably wisely so as his written work was just – only just – adequate, his bent purely practical. I often wondered what happened to him when Enrolled Nurses were phased out.

From Tidworth, and Wroughton, it was quite easy to visit my cousin who lived near Salisbury. One day she took me to the city to visit William Tatton-Brown, an architect, and cousin of hers. It was interesting to meet him, a delightful man, but by then long retired. He was responsible for the demise of Nightingale wards, having advised the government on the design of new hospitals. Nightingale wards had been in all the great hospitals; long, high spaces, with a dozen or more beds on each side, and sister's desk in the middle.

Too late, he found himself a patient in one, at St Thomas's, and subsequently published an apologetic article in the *Nursing Times*. William learnt the camaraderie of these wards; the patients looking out for each other; the central desk enabling staff, especially at night, to keep an eye on everyone. In those days some 'up' patients were well enough to take the early morning tea trolley round, and they would chat to the bedridden, cheering them up.

A scathing article in one nursing journal had painted a ghastly picture of all these people having to live a life of no privacy whatsoever in these circumstances, but the fact was that the lauded four-bed units made caring more difficult. Nowadays of course, the idea of having 'up' patients is long gone. Any patient capable of putting one foot in front of the other – and often not even that – would be sent home pronto. Convalescence is non-existent; the very word, obsolescent. Rapid discharge is said to be desirable in order to avoid the high infection rates in hospitals.

In my day I do not remember such a thing ever being mentioned. Maybe the demise of ward cleaners is to blame. Known as 'Pinks' at King's thanks to their pink uniforms, they worked on a specific ward and were very much part of the ward team. They were loyal and fussy and invaluable, taking a great pride in 'their' ward, and sometimes welcomed as a listener and confidante if patients were too wary of other staff.

Today, all hospital cleaning is delegated to outside contractors. Their staff are given too little time for tasks and none for interaction with patients in wards and departments. Not to mention frequent personnel changes which do not allow familiarity with specific areas. Also, the days of Sister overseeing ward cleaning as well as patient care are gone. Any complaint: 'Send for the cleaning supervisor…'

From Wroughton I had a memorable visit to friends in Spain, thanks to RAF indulgence flights. These were rare, depended on availability of seats, were at short notice and never guaranteed. Also ludicrously cheap – just £6 or £7 for insurance. For one week of leave I hoped to go to Gibraltar. No luck with an indulgence flight, but I went anyway, in February, hoping for some sun. The evening before leaving home I phoned friends Hermione and Sonia in Estepona, to ask what the weather was like. I begged to be forgiven for not going to see them, but explained about the hope for an indulgence flight, which was only to Gibraltar of course. At the time the border into Spain was closed to service personnel, but I just needed a short holiday. 'No problem at all', said Sonia. 'You go down to the marina and find a boat going to Estepona. The going rate is twenty-four pesetas.'

After landing in Gibraltar I called into the RAF Transport office, where a friendly Sergeant also thought 'no problem'. The RAF Golf team was going tomorrow. He wasn't sure if there would be room on the boat for me, but he gave me the Skipper's phone number. I phoned and yes, he could take me.

Next day we sailed from Gib at about 11 am, on a yacht with a husband and wife crew, four golfers, and me. The sun was shining, there was a decent breeze, and I revelled in being on deck. We rounded Europa Point, so over on our left rose the barren, vertical and forbidding face of the Rock. Quite suddenly we appeared to be sailing towards it which was odd … unnecessary … and then not a good idea at all. The crew had become very busy but eventually explained what had happened. The rudder had fallen off! The boat had recently been serviced….

Back round Europa Point help arrived, but wasn't needed. Later we were told by other people that it was only by superb seamanship our crew saved the situation, and got us safely back without assistance. Astonishingly, by teatime we set off again. This time on a much bigger vessel which was home to a family – parents and two small children. Our voyage was uneventful but my arrival was not.

We did not berth in Estepona until 11 pm. Our passports were confiscated until the morning as no immigration officers were on duty, and by the time Customs had finished with us it was nearly midnight. I had intended to walk to El Cobre, but it was well over a mile to the house, which is how I managed to turn up in a taxi, without warning and without any local money, almost in the middle of the night. When I rang the bell the door was opened by a strange woman. It transpired that although I hadn't said I was definitely coming, Hermione and Sonia were sure I would. They had an engagement that evening, but the friend staying with them was charged with answering the phone as they expected a message. The poor lass had an awful cold and had gone to bed early, only to have to get up three times to answer the phone, none of them calls from me. By the time she had to come to the door she was not a happy bunny – and then to be asked to pay the taxi driver…. He hadn't been too happy either; we had to wait quite a while for the door to be answered. Happily, when Hermione and Sonia returned, they thought it was hilarious.

Leaving Estepona wasn't straightforward either. After a great time with the girls, three mornings later they drove me down to the marina, together with several friends. It was touch and go whether we sailed, or so I was led to believe, though not sure how true.

What was true was the swell beyond the harbour; Hermione and Sonia said they would never forget watching our boat bouncing its way out between the harbour walls into the Mediterranean. For me it was huge fun, but they were real land-lubbers. There was a gate on to the sandy beach at the bottom of their garden, with beautiful unspoilt stretches of coast in either direction, but they never went out there, and seemed surprised when I enthused. Sad.

Chapter 16

Germany. Three Separate Postings

1983–1985

WHEN JOINING THE QAs it was obvious that at some point I was likely to be posted to Germany. In 1972 the British military presence there was still huge.

The prospect horrified me as I am so useless at languages, and it always feels rude to be in a civilised country and not speak the lingo. Years later I learnt it is a handicap endured by left-handers; the other side of their brain dominates, making languages difficult. Oh dear, so true.

Not for the first time I was slightly off beat, as it was known that many of my days off were spent at home helping to look after my father. This was a rare commitment for a QA, one senior officer even suggesting that it was my sister's job, despite the fact that she had three small children, and lived twenty miles away. Families were not considered priorities for service personnel, especially single officers.

That said, another senior officer – ambitious, married to a Regimental Colonel, not afraid to make waves and eventually Matron in Chief – kindly offered to see if she could arrange a married quarter so that I could have Daddy with me. Jenny and I were horrified. He might have enjoyed himself, but Germany may not have recovered from the experience. He could be quite a character....

Anyway, ten years after joining the Corps I left Wroughton and drove to Munster. Where I stuck. My four wheels came to a standstill. Despite having driven in Germany before, when I took my father to visit Sue and Peter, friends in Minden, and despite having got myself to Munster, there descended on me an odd and unpleasant fear of driving. The hospital was close enough to the city centre for us to walk there, so it was easy to keep this irrational nonsense to myself. On my first days off, which happened to be a weekend, my only outing was a walk round the perimeter of the hospital – all of a quarter of a mile.

After nearly three weeks I began to pull myself together, and when I left Germany two years later had driven about 40.000 miles. Munster was on the flat North German Plain, but from childhood always wanting views I used to drive to a low ridge of hills where there was a wide, distant sight of the Ruhr. I never did manage to count all the tall industrial chimneys – midgets far away.

Munster itself was pleasant enough, the hospital less so, though it could have been worse. In the Corps there was a widely held perception that midwives refused to work anywhere except in midwifery units but I had proved that not so in my case, with both PSO and Wroughton under my belt. So it would have been possible to request a return to midwifery, where internal rotation was the norm, but I decided not to. Somehow being Sister on the children's ward had seemed OK, but in Munster reality hit.

Terrified of ward sisters throughout my training, and never, ever, wanting to be one myself, now I was really in at the deep end. With a vengeance. Families Ward was the only female ward, so nine consultants had beds. Medical, surgical, gynaecology, dental, ENT, teenagers, you name it.

Military rank as a problem was almost non-existent in the medical services, as care of the patients was paramount. Useless for a Commanding Officer to call out an entire hospital staff on parade. But most doctors, especially consultants, have more, or less, but usually more, well-developed egos. Sister's word absolute? Oh no it isn't.

Complaining to a colleague later, she implied it was my own fault for not managing properly. All I did was name the most difficult consultant physician and she capitulated immediately. An exception to the ego rule, he was a lovely man, no ego whatever, but just impossible. Like most of the main specialists he had three designated beds.

However, he was very kind, and keen to help the many overweight wives, admitting them for a week for low calorie diets. On one notorious

Monday twenty-one women turned up for admission. Any consultant needing an extra bed for some reason could usually borrow from another, as slight flexibility was available. But twenty-one! Needless to say he had exceeded his quota before, but my protests went unheard. He would just go off and see other doctors, and – unbelievably – he got what he wanted time and again. Even with the twenty-one, though how on earth that happened I cannot remember.

The other consultants had their quirks too. Added to all of them the nurses were also unhappy, most of them, especially the juniors. Luckily they settled down fairly quickly. It transpired my predecessor was much disliked and they expected me to be the same. Whether she was a dragon, or difficult, or some other reason, always remained a mystery, but one day a staff nurse enlightened me about the fears of the juniors.

I was well aware of being too easy going, though perhaps fortunate as the best antidote at that time. The ward survived, and so did I, though glad to escape after only five months – to another of the best three months of my life, at HQ BAOR, British Army Of the Rhine, Rheindahlen, near Monchengladbach.

Following that adventure I returned to Munster for three months, so for the sake of continuity will reminisce about Rheindahlen after the end of all the Munster tales. Throughout my posting I went home quite often, usually when on leave. Occasionally, with two weeks' days off added together, I stayed in Germany.

In July I had a memorable trip to Switzerland. By then I had been in Munster four months but still felt rather reluctant to drive, though had managed a few local explorations, taking one or other QA with me. Two of us had a most interesting visit to the Mohne Dam of Dam Busters' fame; my companion was a very nice woman named Judith. She was most comforting when, for the only time ever, I was done for speeding. On the edge of the city we had just left the thirty km sign. The young policeman who stopped me was charming. In English he said 'You were going too fast', spoken with a sympathetic smile. I had failed to notice that after the thirty km derestriction sign a forty km one immediately appeared. Sneaky. Paying the fine was easy, as it could be done in ordinary post offices, but I did not even have to do that as Judith took it for me.

Switzerland was a decidedly last minute decision. Jill, a staff nurse on Families Ward, was going to drive down to Switzerland with her husband for a few days and I told several people of my plan to follow their example. Except that I didn't have a plan, and greatly doubted my willingness to go anywhere.

Telling of my intention was intended to make it more difficult to back out, though with only four days off there was a reasonable excuse for not going so far, but experience had taught me long ago that a long weekend allows immense possibilities...

Only on the day before departure did I decide to go – but not to Switzerland. Just as far as Lake Constance, hoping to at least see Switzerland on the far shore. The drive South went so well that by midday I was almost past Frankfurt, so I stopped to look at a map. A road atlas, actually, of Western Europe. I regret having no memory of which member of the family gave it to me, for it was an invaluable present, in constant use.

The other book worth its weight in gold was my Baedeker's Germany; bought in Blackwells, Oxford, during one of my earliest trips home, and with helpful consequences to this day.

On the face of it just another travel guide, albeit a famous classic, somehow it taught me to look at things properly, noticing details, especially in architecture. It made me realise how much I had missed in the past, particularly when exploring during shore excursions from *Oriana*.

A book that wasn't much help was a BBC one, to use with a tape on a Teach Yourself German Course. Hopeless, though not the fault of the BBC....

I had looked forward to learning French at school but found I could never remember the words. There were no end of short, medium and long language courses available for all army personnel in Germany, from basic ones for squaddies to learn how to order a beer, to long ones for staff working with German colleagues – but not for QAs unless willing to do them during leave. The perennial excuse of not enough staff to cover ward duties etc. Typical.

In the end *Bitte* and *Danke*, please and thank you, had to suffice, with a rare extra word, here and there. However people throughout the country were kind and tolerant, rather to my surprise, and I came to love Germany.

Back with my road map on the A5, I discovered it went in almost a straight line right down to Basel. So even if having barely crossed the border I could honestly claim I had been to Switzerland. In fact, not only did I get as far as Interlaken, I then drove out of town, along the north shore of Lake Thun, to a B&B. It was memorable; a beautiful, classic wooden Swiss house with long balconies hung with geraniums, looking out high over the lake.

The next day I caught the train to the top of the Jungfrau, passing a close-up view of the north face of the Eiger on the way. In bright sunshine I explored the top of the mountain, and from the summit platform watched an avalanche, glad it was some distance away from skiers in the area, as it roared down the side of the long, wide valley below. The skiers just carried on, showing no sign of panic whatever.

Returning to Interlaken the train took a longer route, running below the Eiger, from where there was a view of the entire vast, stark, cut-slice slab of vertical black rock. No wonder it has such a fearsome reputation. To soften the vista, brilliant blue gentians grew at the foot, close to the railway line, in unforgettable beauty.

On another brief expedition I took myself to the Black Forest. Rather disappointing, but Tubingen was a huge bonus. A small, not particularly well-known city, it is built on a steep slope, with a castle at the top, a river at the bottom, and the city square about half way between them. It is a university city, with aspects reminiscent of Oxford, Cambridge, and Durham. Despite many beautiful towns in Germany, Tubingen is my favourite.

These travels from Munster, are not my only memories, as a hospital exercise remains vivid. Before that account, one more expedition; a lift I gave to two girls who wanted to get to Hanover to collect a new car.

After dropping them off I made my way to Celle, an attractive town – and then to Belsen. Now just acres of derelict space, with a few low-key memorials, but the exhibition centre at the entrance gate is awash with horrific photographs. What most impressed me were bus loads of young German soldiers visiting.

It so happened that shortly after that dreadful place, due to two different routes to and from UK ferries, I drove through Ypres and Waterloo. Not just the Menin Gate remains in my memory; the many, many war grave cemeteries of the Somme were mind-boggling. Some were near the main road, but clusters of signposts pointed the way to uncountable others.

In Waterloo I explored both the town and the battlefield. The church in the centre of town had walls lined with memorial tablets, virtually all in English and dedicated to British casualties. In the space of a fortnight Belsen, the Somme and Waterloo. Man's inhumanity to Man.

One day on duty I looked out of a ward window and was very excited to see, in the near distance, an airship. I rushed around telling the staff to come and see. Their reaction? Almost total indifference. I was reduced to pointing out that it was an airship, not a hot air balloon and I had never seen one before. Indeed, did not know any still existed. All a waste of breath, no one interested.

They all had to be interested, or certainly involved, in Maxi-Mash, a major hospital exercise to practice receiving mass casualties. I hated it, barely knowing what I was supposed to be doing, let alone doing it. To make it more realistic everyone slept on floors in unused rooms. Three NCOs were scheduled to share a four bed space with me, but they were so shocked at the idea of sharing with an officer they all disappeared, despite my protests, to I know not where. Now to an infinitely happier posting.

HQ BAOR Rheindahlen

This was the location for the Administration of the British Army of the Rhine. It was near Monchengladbach and also close to the Dutch border. The Big House was exactly that, a vast brick building, rarely seen at its impressive whole, due to a concealing mushroom growth of surrounding satellite buildings – of Nissen hut style, not red brick grandeur.

The senior QA Colonel with responsibility for Corps Admin throughout the British part of Germany had her office there. It barely needs saying that it was not in the Big House itself, but she did live in the Senior Officers' Mess.

I never set foot in the Big House and do not remember anyone who did. QA Majors were attached for three months to learn how Corps admin worked. Most other people had two-year postings, so QAs were a rarity. Only one of us at a time, and we always lived in B mess, one of five large ones for the two or three hundred junior officers. By all accounts QAs were always welcomed although so temporary, and certainly I was.

Thanks to a first class Mess President, and excellent Entertainments Officer, the Mess was a buzzing and happy place.

After only ten days I was being taken to a local shopping centre in a car with four other Mess members, Cathy, a SSAFA sister, and three men. There had already been several social events, and at one point I muttered that B Mess reminded me of Manadon. Instant agreement from one of the men; Terry had been on attachment there. Great place, said he. Indeed! Another incredible coincidence in my life.

At Hallowe'en a Mess party was organised. Only twenty-two of us there, but from the moment it started it fizzed. Dunking for apples had me in one of the teams, despite never having dunked before, and knowing I could not open my eyes under water. To my astonishment I captured an apple at once, so with it in my mouth and blinded by the water, I charged for the back of the team. We won!

But I couldn't see and didn't stop – until I ran full tilt into the grand piano, the edge bashing into my ribs. I was winded; well and truly unable to catch my breath. A horrible experience, it has given me the greatest sympathy for sportsmen and others who suffer such trauma. In the next game, which involved some close contact, I quickly realised more participation would be unwise, so just enjoyed sitting quietly for the rest of the party, enjoying watching the others.

Next day a very straitlaced school teacher told me with disapproval that she heard there was an orgy in B Mess last night. What rubbish! An orgy it was not, just real fun, and an early finish too. The only time I played any Mess games and then only two or three, but the consequences lasted longer.

Coughing was painful for what felt like ages, but stopped at exactly six weeks. Length of time for broken ribs to heal? Six weeks. The pain was never serious enough to send me to a doctor, but if I did not have a fractured rib or two, I have no doubt one was cracked.

The following week our very popular Entertainments Officer was leaving and everyone wanted a great farewell party for her. It was realised that a repeat of Hallowe'en would not work, but sadly neither did the low-key alternative. Nothing made that party spark. Dull, dull, dull. So disappointing, but it convinced me that no matter how much planning and effort goes into organising a party, with the best will in the world the outcome is unpredictable. Success is not guaranteed.

My own record of entertaining was abysmal for thirty years, from the days of cabin 'pour outs' on *Oriana* until I retired from the Corps. All due to what? No idea. The wish for people to relax and enjoy themselves was always there. The nadir was in Berlin, of which more later.

Anyway, the events and pleasant socialising in Rheindahlen B Mess were a joy. Rumour said it was more stodgy than the other four, hard to believe, but all of them had a mix of Corps and Regiments, men and women; plus a few civilians such as school teachers and welfare workers.

For a few weeks B Mess kitchens were closed to allow some major work, (shades of Nepal!) so we all went next door to E Mess for our meals. There did not seem to be quite the same welcoming atmosphere but it was not a problem, and I did like the single, very long dining table. One took the first vacant chair, so could be sitting next to goodness knows who. A whole posse of newly posted-in young officers turned up one week – I think fresh from some high-powered promotion course. At breakfast one morning, on their first day, I sat next to a definitely stressed young man. He managed to relax enough to talk a bit, and confided that in his Regiment no talking at breakfast was the custom.

It transpired he was a Guards Lieutenant. What he thought of joining the Hoi Polloi, let alone sitting next to a woman, goodness knows, nor have I any idea how, or if, he settled down, as our paths never crossed again. Of course in those days women had nothing to do with front line combat, though nurses might not be far behind it.

Following a massive Exercise a huge debrief was held in the lecture theatre. There were some three hundred men in the audience, and five women. Several men were astonished to see me, especially a couple of foreign officers on attachment. Germans I believe, but Dutch, Danish and others were there too.

At one point I had to go to Rinteln to umpire an exercise. The briefing was at midnight, and as I arrived in this enormous garrison, alone, I realised I had no idea of where to go, but somehow arrived in the right place with a minute to spare. Room crowded, no one took the slightest notice of me, then I noticed I was the only woman there. It felt quite odd, which was a surprise.

Details of the actual exercise are remembered only vaguely, with one remark, from Matron, at the end, that I looked ill. Throughout my life more easily tired than many, staying awake for thirty-six hours was not my idea of fun so she was right.

Back in Rheindahlen we had returned to B Mess and most people were delighted, but in our dining room there were tables for six or eight. Friends were astonished when I said I disliked them, much preferring the one long table in E Mess. Arriving in ours, where to sit?

Not to interrupt a couple chatting. Not to butt in on a group already settled. Not to sit alone and look unsociable…. There was surprise, then a chorus of 'You can always join us.' No wonder a happy place.

Apart from all the socialising I spent many days off exploring. Warned to expect extreme cold and snow, it was actually a mild autumn. It was easy to drive to Roermond, in Holland, for Saturday afternoon shopping, when shops in Germany were always closed.

On my first day off, needing washing powder, a successful foray went well until approaching the German check post on returning. No passport – panic; no bother – no one there. I drove straight through.

Much further afield I loved the Eifel, especially the old walled town of Bad Munstereifel. The Moselle; Luxembourg; Aachen; the Rhein Gorge – the latter in November. I sat in an empty car park, close to the water, watching the huge barges, often with a small car aboard. How the traffic lights worked for them was difficult to fathom, but it controlled the narrowest part of the gorge, with a one-way system. High above, the ancient castles on either side, beloved by photographers and illustrators of fairy tales. Later that day, back on the main road, having decided I had gone far enough, I did a U turn. Needless to say, the road was empty, no sign of any other vehicle, but even in November unbelievable on this notoriously busy major highway.

An unusual, great day out was to the Ahr valley during the local wine festival. A German schoolteacher had spent months hoping to find someone to join her. Thanks to a chance remark by a teacher in our Mess, about how disappointed her colleague was, I said I would be happy to go with her – despite only a few days' notice; not the German way of doing things.

Not only is the Ahr valley the most northerly red wine producing area, the wine has an excellent reputation, while the valley itself is beautiful and well worth a visit. We enjoyed a glass of wine in one of the hostelries, and then met a couple who told us we must try some

Feder wine – Feather wine; brand new, only ever available for one week and very special. So we did, and it was absolutely delicious. Tempted to have a second glass, I realised almost instantly that it was extremely alcoholic! Not even many Germans know of it so we were very fortunate to have had it recommended, particularly with such enthusiasm.

The day before this memorable trip with a local civilian German club, I was taken to meet Gilase, the teacher who wanted someone to accompany her. It was the only time I was ever in a German person's home. She lived in a charming, modern flat, furnished with pretty English antiques. A happy visit, and a great bonus as it was a rare privilege.

In between all these socialisings, and many more, I did do some work. Colonel Pease was my boss. We got on well which was a mercy, as there were only the two of us and we were together in her office. Not quite all the time; she would be away on official visits or I would be having liaison tutorials in other areas.

Every month there was a big headache with C340s, the forms from each hospital with a record of staff numbers. The problem was the figures never tallied with the official statistics.... The admin, was quite interesting, but there were too many problems to wrestle with – commonly caused by never enough staff, so it did not appeal to me.

Colonel Pease returned from a home visit to MOD, tasked with finding a Major to be I/C Families ward and also Deputy Matron, in Berlin. After a few days of no one being chosen, somehow I plucked up courage to suggest maybe I could do it.

'Yes,' she said, 'I thought so, and have already told MOD.' Notable that after so long no one else had occurred to either of us, though for all sorts of valid reasons.

In a totally different way Colonel Pease astonished me one day when I opened my post. At home there was a craze for 'head boppers', a toy which was a headband with a couple of stalks sticking up carrying mini windmills. Jenny told me that my niece Alison longed for one but they were sold out everywhere locally, so it was a joy to find one and post it to her. Aged 6, she sent me a lovely thank-you letter, with a drawing of herself running along to make the windmills whirl.

Colonel Pease took one look at it and was extremely impressed, saying at once that Alison had the makings of an artist. She did not explain her reasoning and I did not ask, but I still have the letter and think of Colonel Pease when looking at AliFoxonArt on Facebook or, recently, reading her excellent book on 'Green Sketching'.

There was another adventure – unusual, unexpected but exciting. I drove a train. A WRAC lass from another Mess had driven it, so when by good luck overhearing about this adventure, I thought it surely might be possible for me too…. Enquiries readily led to a visit being arranged. The train was the last surviving military one, an ambulance train, stored in a military depot near Monchengladbach. It was such a vast, open and derelict place, with no signposts, no people, most buildings razed to the ground, no hint of a railway, that I arrived one-and-a-half hours late.

The little railway line, about half a mile long, was out of sight on the far side from the entrance. Despite the awful delay the crew – all two of them, gave me a warm welcome and a comprehensive tour. Externally the carriages looked like conventional rolling stock, but the interiors were an unpleasant surprise.

Short journeys only had been envisaged, just to transport patients from one medical facility to another e.g. Dressing station to Field hospital, or hospital to coast for evacuation. Hence there were three tiers for stretchers on either side, the whole length of the carriage and not much space for anything else. Also, it was impossible to reach patients on the top tier.

There seemed to be no provision for drinks, let alone food, and certainly no sluice for emptying bottles, bedpans, vomit bowls etc. *but*, there was a spacious – comparatively – cabin/office for one. A doctor. Nowhere for nurses, orderlies or other staff. Knowing that patients could be on the train for twenty-four hours – for example being shunted into sidings as vital supplies in freight trains took precedence, I was incensed. No wonder their use was limited, and this last one likely to be scrapped in the not far distant future.

It reminded me of some plans an architect once showed me, for a large new private medical centre. Four large offices for doctors but tiny ones for physios and others; cramped, ridiculous treatment rooms, practical areas and miniscule storage facilities. Actually of course, it is most unfortunate that so many doctors have minimal understanding of what nursing and other ancillary care involves.

After a tour of the carriages we climbed onto the footplate, and after some instruction I was allowed to drive – about a quarter of a mile along the track then back again. It qualified me as a TWIT; in German 'Engine Driver Second Class', and I was given a certificate to prove it.

Before leaving, I had another shock. Beside the line there was a building where all the equipment was stored. Boxes piled high, but a couple with easy access were opened to give me an idea of the contents. The poor men were taken aback by my shocked reaction. There wasn't the slightest semblance of orderly packing, just a chaotic muddle, topped by loose blue capsules. Sodium Amytal three grs; strong barbiturates, thrown over the chaos indiscriminately. The crew were unconcerned and I strongly suspect that my plea to collect them all and put under lock and key was ignored.

After Christmas leave at home I had another ten days in Rheindahlen before leaving with a heavy heart to return to Munster. However, on the last day before most people dispersed for Christmas leave, it was decreed that everyone in B Mess would have breakfast together. In pyjamas and dressing gowns. I was not very bothered at being last to arrive, after going to an early service in chapel, only to be greeted with some relief, and escorted to sit next to the Mess President. Startling!

At the end of the meal he stood up and made a speech. Then the penny dropped. I was being dined out.

With many folks posted in on short attachments, the custom was that only those there for a full two years would be dined out The QAs, only ever there for three months, were so well liked that they were the exception and always honoured, being presented with a tile with a picture of the Big House as a memento. In memory of my collision with the grand piano I was also given a mouth organ as a grand piano was felt to be too large. After this accolade I had to make a speech. *Quelle horreur*.

When leaving Wroughton, by an unheard of stroke of dreadful bad luck, I was the only person being dined out at that particular dinner. Normally it was two or more people, and only the senior person spoke. But I was landed. Army in an RAF Mess, and a female to boot. Ouch! At least I had advance warning. Luckily inspiration came to me when doing some ironing. The outcome was short, well received and I survived.

So in Rheindahlen, to give myself a few seconds to think before replying, I started by saying that when I was dined out in Wroughton I had thought of something to say while doing some ironing. Instantly a voice called out, 'I've got some ironing you could do, Mary.'

I duly went to Munster and there are just a couple of amusing mini incidents to record from that time, both connected with Irish Guards, hospital neighbours up the road in Oxford Barracks.

At some official but non-uniform party, with German guests, one man chatted to a group of us in impressive English. Fluent and impeccable, I was full of admiration. Later I discovered that this 'German gentleman' was actually the CO of the Irish Guards... Doubtless he was at his most fluent on 17 March, St Patrick's Day.

The Battalion's Colonel in Chief, the Queen Mother, always joined the celebrations, to present shamrocks to the soldiers and to meet the families and guests. Stevie, a QA, was to be the on-the-hoof blood supply for Her Majesty if needed. As one of the guests she was to wear civilian clothes, including a hat – but she did not own one. Not surprising; hats had been out of fashion for years.

However, Princess Diana had hit the scene by then, and I owned a cerise, side-tilted straw hat similar to one of her styles, bought for attending a military celebration back at home. My friends Sue and Peter had invited me to the presentation of new Colours to the Duke of Wellington's Regiment. (The Duke of Boots.) On arriving for a curry lunch on the second day of the celebrations, young subalterns were greeting the guests, taking their coats etc., and one of them took my hat and put it on. It suited him, he looked terrific, but of course suffered much ribbing from his fellows. Stevie borrowed this titfer with a history – and was introduced to HM, so my hat met the Queen Mother.

And once upon a time my service cap went to Buckingham Palace for a medal presentation; another loan – this time when the owner's own hat was thought too old and unfit for meeting Royalty.

Before leaving Munster the ward staff took me out for a meal. Not a particularly united crowd, I expected a rather dull evening, but how wrong I was. It proved the opposite. A fun, cheerful, get together, with lots of laughter, especially over a bowl of ice cream. It was monstrous. The biggest of the cafe's speciality ices, one of the girls had long wanted to try it, but the reality was huge and ridiculous. When it was put in front of her, we all fell about laughing. Four of her friends helped her to eat it.

To my astonishment, at the end of the evening they gave me a present. A Lladro figure of a tall, slim girl with a basket in one hand

and a chicken cradled in the crook of her other arm. From that night on called The Munster Girl, and loved ever since.

She came from a shop in East Berlin, bought by one of our staff nurses during a recent visit. Most Lladro pieces are Spanish, but apparently a second Lladro brother settled in East Germany, less famous, but similar work and very good. Normally I'm not too keen on Lladro figures, but my girl is graceful, beautiful and very special.

Berlin

Getting to Berlin involved crossing the East/West German border, then a sixty mile 'corridor' through East Germany into the city via another border control. Most people thought the German border far nastier than the Berlin one, which was true, for the city was far more low key.

From the West side of the East border, after passing through a wire fence the road wound half a mile across no-man's-land, an empty area almost devoid of plant life, let alone anything else. It had an eerie, evil atmosphere. 'You're very hot on atmosphere, Mary', my Rheindahlen boss once told me. At the far end, beyond a second fence, one parked the car and went into a small roadside building. Inside was a windowless lobby, with doors left and centre, a blank, closed hatch on the right. Silence. At the bottom of the hatch – which looked unopenable – was a letter box slot into which one slid the all-important travel document. It disappeared, taken by an unseen hand. Spooky. Silence. Stand and wait. Document appeared back through slot.

Onward. The corridor road was ordinary, in fact uninteresting, enclosed by trees apart from, rarely, the blank wall of a house. Minimal traffic. Two hours allowed for the journey, and stopping permitted, so I pulled into a lay-by for a quick picnic coffee, subsequently discovering most people disliked the corridor, some intensely, and could never wait to complete it, so I never admitted to my coffee stop.

Here I may as well complete the tales of my other corridor experiences, though the ones going home for Christmas leave and back were entirely straightforward, including the usual travel document. Hannelore was responsible for them. She was a German woman in the hospital Admin Office; had worked with the British since 1949, and was much loved.

In typical German fashion she was meticulous, and exceptionally fussy about the Corridor Travel Permit.

She knew tales of drivers turned back due to a missing comma, let alone a spelling mistake. For some forgotten reason my final departure was postponed by one day, then, regretfully, goodbye Berlin. Not stopped at the city checkpoint, at the far end of the corridor I went into the surreal building and posted my document in the usual way, and waited. And waited. And waited. Someone else came in, posted his document, had it returned, and departed. Still I waited. Suddenly one of the doors opened! A young officer came out with my permit in his hand, and said something in German which I didn't understand. Then he indicated the date. Wrong one! It was for the day before, I was supposed to have travelled, though a new permit had been done for me. Really shocked, I said – in English of course – that I would go back at once.

To my astonishment he said *nein, nein*, and indicated that I could leave and continue my journey, though at our own checkpoint I must ask for the correct date to be inserted. He even smiled! Once again no-man's-land felt eerie and unpleasant, so it was cheering to arrive at our British checkpoint. There the police were amazed at my request; it was obviously unheard of....

To return to my time in Berlin....

In Germany, and Cyprus, QA Majors had a sitting room and separate bedroom; in Munster and Cyprus, sharing a bathroom with just one other person. In Berlin, everyone had their own bathroom and the accommodation was quite famous, regularly lauded by people who had been there. So many people had told me I would love the rooms in Berlin that finding them pretty awful was a shock

The sitting room was enormous and dreadfully dark, as the big window was shadowed by a wide, ugly, solid concrete balcony. Grossly under furnished, it was impossible to create a comfortable atmosphere. Also endlessly noisy, because although both rooms looked out to a stretch of grass and thick belt of tall trees, the twelve-lane Heerstrasse, a main Berlin thoroughfare, ran nearby. SO noisy! It was only ever quiet for about half an hour in the early hours, around 2 am.

The bathroom was another disappointment. All the rooms in Munster were light and sunny, including the bathroom, but here it was an internal, windowless one, made worse by showing its age, with well-worn fittings which made me long for the fresh ones I had just left. Usually it took me about forty-eight hours to settle in a new Mess; here, ten days.

I decided to give a coffee party in the big sitting room. Since *Oriana* days, as previously mentioned, there was something of a jinx on my efforts at entertaining, but this party was on a level of its own. What follows is an exact copy of what I wrote straight afterwards – though omitted noting that all 'proper' coffee in Germany is excellent. They say we do not spend enough on it in the UK, so the quality is not always good.

Gaelic Coffee Eighteen Guests.

June Humphries and Stevie Webster asked to help, to overcome party jinx.

June didn't come due to a meeting. It was cancelled but she cried off anyway.

Stevie ill and only stayed ten minutes.

All the guests arrived at once, on the dot of 8.30 pm.

First one asked for a beer, which I had not planned for.

I had wine but forgot it – found in fridge later.

I wasn't quite ready – cream not in jug – but it was sour anyway.

Someone sat on the sofa, which had been mended the day before after months with a broken castor shaft. It broke again.

So accustomed to instant Gold Blend I never thought of doing percolated ground coffee.

Guests disdainful.

Then the fuses blew. No light, no music, no kettle.

By all the laws the rest of the party should have been great. It wasn't.

It was stodgy beyond belief – and had rather an unpleasant undercurrent of critical dissatisfaction.

'Sit down for five minutes' said my most unwelcome guest, as I tried frantically to cope with demands for second coffees before everyone had been served with their first.

The biggest man sat on the smallest stool and fidgeted + +, while Joe D. sat on the other small one and looked silly, while chairs stayed empty.

Thankfully most Berlin memories are far happier. But reading this sorry tale again, the cream – 'It was sour anyway' – still makes me laugh. It summed up the entire fiasco.

BMH was purpose built, including a complete hospital underground, near Hitler's infamous 1936 Olympic Stadium. It was there that black American Jesse Owens won four gold medals. Hitler behaved appallingly, refusing to shake Owens' hand, let alone present the medals, his belief in Aryan supremacy demonstrably scuppered.

It was great to be in the city in 1984 when, with a big ceremony, the road between the hospital and the stadium was renamed Jesse-Owens-Allee. Unable to be there for the actual ceremony, later it was a joy to see the new finger post street name sign, still decorated with a pretty floral garland wound around it.

The stadium and the hospital were in the suburb of Charlottenburg, an old and pleasant part of Berlin some distance from the city centre. The Schloss Charlottenburg was my favourite building in the entire city, East or West, a long, low yellow palace with a pretty central dome. It housed a Meissen museum full of beautiful porcelain.

In the opposite direction one soon reached the woods and water of the Grunewald and the River Havel, both attractive and frequently visited. The extraordinary thing was exploring further, discovering that West Berlin covered a huge area inside the Wall, including agricultural land. One Sunday afternoon I drove sixty miles, but had only covered about a quarter of the massive modern suburbs and open country of fields and farming.

In another suburb, Dahlem, I went to see a thatched U-Bahn station. There I found a place called Domäne Dahlem – a sort of commune – where they were having an open weekend festival. Small animals; sheep-shearing demonstration; blacksmith; stalls; lots of fun. Next day

I returned, taking one of the girls with me, and we ate potato pancakes, classic German food, here cooked on top of an old oil drum and the best I ever tasted anywhere.

That rather sums up Berlin. No end of interesting places to see and unexpected things to do, as well as myriad musical, theatrical and other events provided for entertainment.

One memorable expedition was a flight right round the Wall, in an RAF helicopter. RAF Gatow was a small airfield out in the country and right beside the Wall. It had an excellent shop, where I bought my Dresden boy and girl figures.

Three outstanding memories of Berlin include two in the East, but the other was in a small, unremarkable Egyptian museum in an ordinary street in the West. The main, huge, impressive one had been bombed, and though partially reopened it was over in the East and rescued pieces remained in the West.

The exhibits were small, interesting on the whole but with one outstanding, world famous treasure; the head of Nefertiti. She sat alone in a free-standing glass case, in the middle of the gallery, at eye level for anyone of average height. My friend Helen, visiting Berlin, had wanted to go there. As I had been before I stood for a while beside Nefertiti. All of a sudden I had such a surreal moment that I have been ever grateful for corroboration.

Sideways on to me, a young couple were strolling along in the aisle beyond in the most ordinary way imaginable. Unimaginably, the man's profile was identical to Nefertiti.

Same shape of head, same profile, same colouring – just the same. It was ridiculous, it couldn't be – but I managed to alert Helen and she agreed at once. He was so normal and unremarkable – and doubtless never knew, because neither Helen nor I felt confident enough to attract his attention and try to explain.

It was almost impossible for civilians to cross into East Berlin, but the Allied Forces – British, American and French, were encouraged to go; 'exercising their democratic right'. Once through Checkpoint Charlie there were no specific boundaries except in one or two small areas, e.g., near admin buildings. There were, however, unwritten rules about not straying too far. The only time I remember venturing away from the immediate city centre was when a doctor took a few of us to visit a Holocaust Museum. Small, but extremely evocative. Evil. Nasty. A reminder of Belsen.

In the centre itself there was plenty to see, including the vast, partially reopened museums on Museum Island. Above all there was the Opera. Within a week of being posted in, I not only went to the opera but did the driving, taking three passengers, on a trip planned and known about before I left Munster.

I do not remember the opera at all, but joyfully recall parking in the almost deserted Unter den Linden. A wonderful experience, with the scent of the lime blossoms unforgettable. In those days this wide, famous Strasse culminated in a dead end, at the Brandenburg Gate.

There were certain restaurants where we were assured of a welcome and good food. One filled the top level of a twenty-two storey tower block. Going there was considered slightly more venturesome than anywhere else, because it was known to be patronised by East German hierarchy. On one occasion some British would-be diners were turned away due to some big official party taking place.

Although I was dined out in the Mess before leaving I was also taken for a meal in the East, and this time we were welcome. A large group, about twenty of us. We were given one long table at the far end of the big room. That was the night I ventured to try smoked eel and found it was delicious; remarkably similar to smoked salmon. At the end of the meal of course, came the reckoning. Everything in East Berlin was paid for in cash; East German Deutschmarks. Very cheap.

Gradually I became aware of an odd undercurrent, first among a few men at the far end, then working down the length of the table and involving everyone. Eventually I learnt the problem. Not enough money. As I was the guest I had, most unusually, not taken any cash with me, so could not help. After twenty minutes of increasingly frantic calculating, and increasing speculation about our fate, we could see the waiters getting worried too, but at last enough cash was gathered and all was well.

A lovely evening with a decidedly hairy ending! This incident could have ended with considerable difficulty, but the other potential problem was brief and very different. It happened at Checkpoint Charlie.

A place of misery, with even an exceptionally nasty murder in the early years, it was the sole crossing place between East and West

Berlin after the Wall was built. First an American guard post, then the road became a no-man's-land with chicanes for several yards, then the East German guard post. It had been erected at speed and in secrecy, appearing almost complete in one night; intended to stop the haemorrhage of East Germans fleeing the Communist regime. By 1983 it remained unaltered since its opening, depressing to see, and with a grim atmosphere which made all of us glad to complete the crossing, in either direction, the US guards as unsmiling as the German ones. Our cars all had special number plates and uniforms had to be worn always, so sometimes we were just waved through. One evening I drove our Matron in Chief, Brigadier Rooke to the opera, together with the senior QA Colonel in BAOR and our own matron. We were all in Mess Dress, our long grey and scarlet evening dresses; worn without service hats, and when needed, non-uniform coats were allowed – often fur jackets in those days real. Or fake, like mine.

When we stopped at the East barrier the guard, an older man, looked puzzled, then put his head in the window and asked for identification. Quite right, no sign of any uniforms. Sitting beside me, the Brigadier said nothing, but quietly eased her jacket off her shoulders. On her epaulettes, in addition to her Brigadier rank three stars and a crown, at the edge were the brass letters QHNS; Queen's Honorary Nursing Sister. This entitled her to the gold aiguilettes she wore on one shoulder. She also has several medals; the QA one we all wore, plus a couple of service ones and her RRC Royal Red Cross, awarded for outstanding service.

On seeing all this emblazoned glory the guard's jaw dropped. He stepped back, stood to attention, gave a smart salute – then burst out laughing. So did we. An abiding memory of a happy experience at an unhappy spot.

Checkpoint Charlie was not the only place of ghastly past atrocities in Berlin, but by the time I was there tensions had eased a little and it was a dynamic city which I loved.

Almost forgotten – despite thinking it would never be forgotten – a train journey to Venice, starting from Berlin in the American overnight military train to Frankfurt. Exciting three days exploring the beautiful Queen of the Adriatic.

All these tales of Berlin, but I haven't yet mentioned work!

As in all hospitals there were staffing problems, especially on my Families Ward. Which was odd, because our BMH, being an isolated special case, was always maintained by MOD with a full establishment.

When Matron (with whom I got on very well) was away I worked down in her office, which included wrestling with the notorious C340, this time from the opposite end to HQ BAOR. It was while doing this that the penny dropped about my own ward. Built on the race track principle, it had two and four bedded rooms and sister's office round the outside, an inner core with bathrooms, sluice, sterilising room etc., and a corridor running right round between the two.

In the far-side corner from my office, and so invisible, was a small, designated children's unit. Under no circumstances was it to be left without at least one nurse there, and usually two. In effect, it meant two wards to be staffed, not one. No wonder there were problems. Having tumbled to this discrepancy did I tell anyone, let alone make a fuss? No. In the past, if I protested – rare indeed – I was shot down instantly. No matter that my complaint might be valid, it suggested a troublemaker; not to be tolerated. Presumably in the twenty years or so since the hospital was established, no one had noticed the one / two ward dilemma. If it worked for twenty years who was I to rock the boat?

It reminds me of the other time I kept quiet, a year or two later.

When at the Queen Elizabeth Military Hospital Woolwich in 1985 I was asked if I would like to be in the QA contingent at the Festival of Remembrance in the Royal Albert Hall. No thank you! I turned it down flat. Chiefly because it was impossible to imagine myself coping with marching down those steps – despite knowing everyone was trained and rehearsed meticulously by a Guards Sergeant Major.

However, there was another reason, about which I never said a word. The Festival largely involved other ranks and junior officers. Participation by Captains, let alone Majors, tended to be as rare as hens teeth, and it bothered me that the QAs would be perceived as over-promoted by watching hierarchy. But I was not the one to point this out. A quiet word with someone senior might have worked, but it seemed unlikely and I kept quiet.

A brief aside about the Berlin budget. To impress the East money was poured into the West, often paying for cultural events such as visits by the Royal Shakespeare Company and world class musicians.

Once a month a very senior member of NAFAS (National Association of Flower Arranging Societies), would be flown in from the UK, and a one-and-a-half hour demonstration would be given in a hall near the hospital. There was a huge and excellent covered flower market in the city, but absolutely no greenery was available. The demonstrators would arrive with long flower boxes filled wit greenery, then, while talking non-stop, create half a dozen widely differing displays. Their skill was riveting and their beautiful work, plus left over bits, were given away at the end via a draw organised through raffle tickets.

The talks and explanations were fascinating; one speaker reminisced about helping with the flowers, when young, at Queen Elizabeth's wedding in 1947. Too bad I only attended three, not having heard of them earlier. They were not just for hospital staff of course; many wives from units all over Berlin enjoyed them.

Two widely varying aspects of my life as a QA came sharply into focus during this time. First, 'proper' nursing.

For some strange reason I spent an evening on the men's ward, though in fact just looking after four women in a separate room. They had all had major dental surgery that day, and on my own I settled them for the night, with routine post-op care. Bedpans; bowls for hands and face washes; op gowns off and nighties on; drinks; mouth washes; analgesia; pillows plumped and made comfortable; lights dimmed and call bells within reach. The kind of care scarcely changed since I might have been doing it as a student nurse thirty years before.

Long afterwards it dawned on me that it had been my last ever totally practical ward nursing. I still have happy recollections of a calm, rewarding evening – because there was enough time to do everything properly. If only it were ever thus. Nowadays the patients would not only be up to the loo, but probably on their way home. The second aspect couldn't have been much further removed from the first – attending a court martial.

Two non-legal members attend the court, with specific remits which include passing verdicts of Guilty or Not Guilty. (Serious cases would be dealt with back in the UK.) Called to attend one day, in my pressed and tidy No.2 suit, with black court shoes (of which more later), I walked from the nearby hospital up to the large, imposing building which housed UK HQ Berlin. Originally the Admin centre for the 1936 Olympics, the

151

courtroom was in there; a huge, high, impressive room, with a layout more or less identical to any courtroom at home.

It was daunting to sit on the dais facing everyone, only the President, and Judge Advocate on the dais with us, the Junior and Senior representative non-legal members. The junior member was a very young male officer. In my topsy turvy career I had never been a member of a court martial, let alone a Senior member, but there I was, the Senior…

The case was sad, involving a physical assault which happened to a much loved family member for no obvious reason – that it happened was not in dispute. All I wanted to know was: Why?

Eventually the President, a Colonel, asked for my verdict. Oh dear. This threw me into a dilemma. Procedural rules dictated that the Junior Member should be asked first, and it would have been useful if he had been first, as his verdict would have been interesting and possibly even helpful,

I had no idea whether I was being asked as courtesy to a lady, or tested to find out if I knew the correct routine. However it was not a time to quibble, the atmosphere was far too formal. Guilty. I left feeling sad, having helped to send a man to prison.

Women were only just beginning to be appointed to Courts Martial, and courtesy from senior officers to QAs was quite common in those days, so probably wrong of me to suspect them trying to catch me out. Which brings me to the shoes.

For several years it was well nigh impossible to buy plain black court shoes to wear with No.2 uniforms. They all had gold trim of one sort or another. Rarely needed, I had survived without any for ages, but for the Court Martial a pair was essential. I was lucky to find one, though horribly expensive and with slim, almost stiletto heels which were too high. They worried me, but with care I was able to walk in them, and was approaching HQ on the last day in court when the Brigadier appeared some distance ahead. He of the fearsome reputation – the last person I wanted to meet. He saluted, which was a puzzle as I could not see anyone else, but surely he would not be saluting me? Even if my legs did look longer than usual. When he was closer, within normal saluting distance, I saluted him and said 'Good Morning, Sir.' He returned my salute, but with a bit of a cynical smile. He was not the only higher rank officer to salute me; it was an acknowledgement in the same style as they would greet wives, daughters or friends. I was also kissed goodbye by two Commanding Officers at my farewell interviews when being posted. Doubtless women today would be horrified by this, but it was a different time.

To me it was a happy era in the Forces; the deadness of formality relaxing a little, giving way to some friendly reactions, without, in my experience, ever any sexual insinuations. Or maybe it was because I was older and already grey-haired, so no threat, because I did not become a QA until I was 34 – nearly too old to join, and never quite became indoctrinated in military attitudes.

Perhaps they would be even more upset by a group of RAMC doctors to whom a mention of Florence Nightingale was like a red rag to a bull. A few QAs were with this group when a casual reference to Flo was made, with a quite startling effect. Clearly her excoriating reports regarding the conditions in the military hospital in the Crimea still rankled over a century later. Again, women today would be horrified by this, but while senior ranks had to be saluted by juniors first and would then return the courtesy, junior RAMC doctors (i.e. Captains), would never dream of saluting a lady QA Major.

My hesitant reactions to the Brigadier's salute, and to the President of the court requesting my verdict first, are summed up in one word: Inept. A word I feel applied too often in my career, and how I survived for thirty-eight years, or the profession survived me, remains an unsolvable mystery.

My last three postings, to Queen Elizabeth Military Hospital, Woolwich; Princess Mary's RAF Hospital, RAF Akrotiri, Cyprus; and finally the Cambridge Military Hospital Aldershot, did only a little to dispel this impression.

It was a relief to retire, my QA days ending not with a bang but a whimper. 'Retirement is heaven' I once said to my brother-in-law, to his considerable surprise. 'Oh, I didn't know', he replied. Why should he? All the times I forgot things, reacted stupidly or not at all, were best kept to myself when possible.

I knew the standards I aspired to, but did not always achieve. At least I only left a patient on a bedpan once – and my adventures off duty were unsurpassable.

Mention of a lifetime of adventures in my off duty makes me realise Cyprus should not be disposed of in one word, so here goes....

Chapter 17

Cyprus
1985–1987

MY POSTING CAME as a shock. An unwelcome one; instantly, and instinctively, I knew I didn't want to go. As this was a plum posting, it seemed an odd reaction.

The news first came via a phone call in April 1985, from the MOD. Colonel Pease, my boss in Rheindahlen, now in London, wondered if I would consider going to Cyprus at the end of the year? A kind, thoughtful gesture; she was aware that I was still helping to look after my father. Despite misgivings I said yes at once.

The job description was slightly strange, because I would be the senior QA in Cyprus and Deputy Matron in Akrotiri, but neither title acknowledged on paper nor by word of mouth, (Nor, it transpired, in any meaningful action.) Being the senior QA was almost a non-job. Being a senior QA in Princess Mary's RAF Hospital was more than the RAF could stomach, and anyway I was to be I/C Outpatients so that was enough for all official lists etc.

All seemed well with various arrangements for help with care for my father by the time I flew from Brize Norton to Akrotiri on 12 December 1985. Many people had commiserated with the thought of a posting so near Christmas to a new place where, knowing no one, the socialising would be difficult. In practice, invitations flowed in to ensure that I felt included, and I was welcomed to all sorts of events and parties. It was a happy crash course in getting to know people.

RAF Akrotiri covered much of the southern Cypriot Akrotiri peninsula, and was accessed from the rest of the island by only one road.

154

Accommodation blocks, married quarters and workshops were scattered over a huge area, with the runway down one side.

My block was only shared with one other person, a Princess Mary's Royal Air Force Nursing Service Squadron Leader, on the opposite side of the patch where Matron had her own block. Both were isolated down a long footpath to our gardens, with playing fields beyond the garden fence and hedge. The bonus was being nearer the Officers' Mess than anyone else, just a short walk through the gardens. These were at best, rather arid, but a great joy in the spring was seeing anemones appear – scattered single stems with different coloured blossoms. Biblical Lilies of the Field, a lovely surprise.

My sitting room had a door out on to the veranda, the bedroom behind it, and a passage parallel to the veranda linking the kitchenette/laundry and bathroom with my neighbour, Yvonne Mapp. Yvonne was an unusual and interesting person, having come over from the West Indies to train as a nurse she stayed in the UK, despite having no family members this side of the Atlantic.

Very quiet but sharply intelligent, she soon became a friend, and then a close and precious one. We both had difficulties at work so it was immensely cheering to be able to discuss our problems and support each other. More than thirty years later she was still a valued and special friend, so her death in 2021 was a sad blow.

Off duty opportunities were myriad and varied beyond measure. They included exploring Roman ruins and ancient Greek Orthodox monasteries, walking in the Troodos mountains, or skiing in the winter (though not for me), swimming from our own beaches or others, and often enjoying meals and local wine in village tavernas.

Concerts and Shakespearean plays in the Roman amphitheatre at Curium were special treats, not least when a full moon just above the sea formed the backdrop. Magical.

A number of British civilians belonged to the Limassol Amateur Dramatic Society. They did an annual Shakespeare production at Curium, the play during my time being an excellent production of *Much Ado About Nothing*. More than twenty years later I enthused about it to a new neighbour, John Colston. John and his wife had retired from Cyprus to the Isle of Seil, where I now live, and he was astonished that

I had seen the production – I was astonished that he had produced it. To prove that we were talking about the same production, the next day I popped the programme through his letterbox, complete with his name as producer. Sometimes being a hoarder is useful!

Another memorable evening at Curium was a concert given by the Western RAF band. Good music, good vocals, good solos, good fun, with Princess Alexandra as the guest of honour. HRH was directly in my line of sight, and for the entire evening she sat bolt upright without appearing to move. Royal training. She was in Akrotiri to visit the hospital because she was – and in 2024 still is – Patron of Princess Mary's Royal Air Force Nursing Service. Before she arrived everyone was asked if they had ever met her previously.

At the start of her hospital tour the CO brought the Princess to his office to introduce five of his senior staff. She bounced in asking if she had met any of us before, no doubt having done her homework, but when I said, 'Yes, in Australia in 1967', her reaction was unexpected. 'Are you sure?' she said. Then after a moment added, 'You're absolutely right!'

HRH and her husband Angus Ogilvy had been staying with the Governor General at his home on the shore of Sydney Harbour, directly opposite Circular Quay. Apparently the Princess had looked out of a window and, seeing *Oriana*, the ship she had launched in 1960, berthed there, exclaimed: 'That's my ship!' A visit on board was promptly arranged. I hope she enjoyed seeing the large, beautiful portrait of herself, hanging on the wall between the two entrances to the first class lounge, named the Princess Room.

It was a private visit which she had all but forgotten. Amazed at the recollection, she went on to say that the visit hadn't been entirely successful – it had not been altogether approved. I remember having read somewhere, long before we met in Akrotiri, that her 1967 visit to Australia had earned her a telling off, though I've no idea why. I am as certain as can be that it was on the tip of her tongue to explain, but her training in discretion kicked in and she changed her intended remark into a bland one about a return visit in 1978, an official visit that went well. Too bad.

When thinking about what to write about Cyprus the list grows ever longer. So many things were astonishing to some degree or other, but one decision was quickly made. Nothing about work to be included. Not difficult, as much has been obliterated from my memory and there is little in my diary about a variety of problems. Early after being posted in, I made a conscious decision not to record them. That said, there are just a couple of work related tales.

An official visit to the small army hospital in Dhekelia, which included a maternity unit, was arranged shortly after I was posted in. Go by car? Government transport or drive myself? No, the RAF would fly me the eighty miles there by helicopter. Hence I arrived in uniform, complete with briefcase, at 84 Squadron, to be greeted by mild consternation as they were not expecting me. Not a great problem; within five minutes my name was added to the manifest. The flight was grand – sitting beside an open door, enjoying the terrain below, including noticing some Roman ruins never subsequently identified.

The other on-duty tale is two pronged. For some unremembered reason the family beaches had been closed for some time, but reopened for August Bank Holiday. That Sunday afternoon many families were enjoying the sea when terrorists lobbed a couple of bombs over the fence, aimed at the nearby runway. There were no planes there on a Sunday and although virtually no damage was achieved, two mums on the beach were slightly injured and brought to TPMH. I was duty matron so much involved. The next morning the mums had been awake much of the night, one extremely proud of her 8-year-old daughter, who had thrown a towel over a 2-year-old's head and led him to the clubhouse.

The news hit the headlines in the UK and the press wanted to interview the casualties. I said not today; they still needed rest, but could be interviewed tomorrow. Well of course that did not suit press immediacy at all, nor did it suit RAF PR – always far more active than the Army or Navy. Consequently the press arrived in droves.

Hearing a noise in the main corridor I looked out on to a most surreal sight. A caterpillar of human legs tramping past. It took a couple of seconds to register the cause of this bizarre spectacle. Every man was carrying a huge camera on his shoulder, so big it concealed head and torso completely. I do wish I had a photo of them.

Subsequently the little girl's mother, who revelled in the publicity and was annoyed with me for suggesting a delayed interview, had her daughter appear on TV as one of the Children of Courage that year.

Meanwhile the authorities (who months later admitted they had grossly overreacted), among other measures put a twenty-four-hour guard on the hospital main gate. Never mind that it was three miles away from the main station, totally isolated at the end of a single track open road, easily visible across open 'bondu' (low scrubland). Never mind that the hospital was situated at the point of a triangle, with the sea and jagged rocks on two sides. Never mind that the Geneva Conventions prohibits attacks on hospitals – though perhaps that is unknown or disregarded by terrorists and therefore irrelevant.

All that said, guards at the gate were, frankly, ridiculous. Nevertheless, guards at the gate there were, with nurses soon roped in as the rosters could not be filled otherwise. Combat kit, complete with boots, had to be worn despite temperatures in the 90s Fahrenheit.

Someone remarked that the nurses should wear interrupted pattern (camouflage) bikinis. In the middle of all this it was my job to reconcile nursing rosters with guard-duty rosters. Irreconcilable due to lack of staff – but try to explain that to anyone who is not a nurse administrator.

One of the first things I needed to arrange on arrival in Cyprus was acquiring a car. Apart from the distance from our quarters in the main Station area, the staff bus times were no use when duty matron, or for others with on call times.

The local garages had all of us sewn up, offering small cars for juniors, mid-range for people like me and bigger, posher ones for senior officers. Paperwork was expedited and I was soon the owner of a Mazda 323. It served me well, including driving through Europe when posted home, but first enabled endless exploring in Cyprus.

Shocking boasting, but a puff for women drivers. On Easter Monday REME (Royal Electrical and Mechanical Engineers) organised a big car rally. Matron and I were invited to join as guests.

As navigator, Rowena was so useless at map reading that I had to stop the car three times to find our way around a tangle of back streets through industrial Limassol. However, at the checkpoints there were quiz questions etc., and at the final one we were handed one of those little toy plastic frames filled with jumbled up tiles in all but one space. Rowena whizzed them around and made a complete picture in seconds. For her it had been a favourite childhood game with her brother. Her expertise impressive, her non-existent navigational ability redeemed.

When the results were announced a rather puzzled voice said winner, 'a Mary Sandilands'. (Who she?) A gold cup recently donated was nabbed by Rowena, with no hint of sharing. Never mind, each of us received a small wooden shield. Winner inscribed on a metal map of Cyprus and an additional plate at the base engraved with event, date and my name.

Of course, as guests – let alone as women – it was beyond tactless of us to win, and publicity was worse than low key, it was non-existent. However, one man was delighted for us, and determined to arrange a photograph. With difficulty he coordinated our availability with that of an official photographer, but we never saw any of his photographs.

To make matters worse, though I have no idea whether REME knew or not, three days earlier, on Good Friday, I had won an IAM manoeuvring competition. Despite the best efforts of the judge, who docked more points than he should have done. Interestingly he was one of the IAM instructors, and our previous Matron had commented that she thought he didn't like women and I had agreed. He was a man of very small stature, with a giant of a wife who had a forbidding expression. We wondered how much that might be something to do with it.

Despite dozens of interesting places I visited in Cyprus, two stand out in my memory.

The first is Cape Gata, on the south-eastern tip of the Akrotiri peninsula. Few folk went there, it was quite a long drive, though still part of the Station. Just a small, flat, grassy piece of land, with a shallow little sandy bay on one side and a low but lethal rocky shore facing the Mediterranean. The small bay opened into the enormous Episkopi Bay, with Limassol distant at the far end backed even more distantly by the Troodos mountains. Peaceful and beautiful, I loved it

Also beautiful was Kyrenia, a picture-postcard little harbour in northern Cyprus, the Turkish part of the island. The Blue Line, patrolled by UN soldiers, maintained a closed border between there and the Greek part of Cyprus, but a crossing for us was possible at a checkpoint in Nicosia. One arrived with fingers crossed, because it could be closed at any time, or passage refused, without warning or explanation.

Once through, Kyrenia was only a twenty-five minute drive beyond, so day trips were feasible. It was also possible to include a short drive then steep climb up to fairy tale St Hilarion castle, Crusader built on the edge of a cliff, with a steep dizzying drop below on the seaward side. In the small museum in ugly Kyrenia castle – its long curtain wall edged the far side of the harbour – was a 4,000-year-old boat excavated from about a mile offshore by an American archaeologist. It was in an amazing state of preservation and so were a number of large amphorae which carried a cargo of almonds. Thousands of nuts had been salvaged and some were scattered around at random. They were extraordinary, because they looked as if they might have come from the market a day or two ago.

There is no doubt the boat deserved world-wide recognition, but it was said to remain unknown because the man who rescued it never wrote it up or published any details in archaeological or other professional journals. He had been urged to by one or two people over a long period of time, but died without doing so. A shame, for it is one of the most memorable things I have ever seen in a museum. I was lucky enough to go to Kyrenia several times, and even stayed overnight once, with Yvonne, as permitted three times a year.

A privilege I was extremely fortunate to enjoy was attending a traditional Cypriot wedding. It could be argued I was there thanks to Archbishop Makarios. He had been touring a hospital when he met a 19-year-old boy who had been an inpatient for three years, following a bad motorcycle accident. The Archbishop arranged for him to be sent to Headley Court, the famous RAF Rehabilitation centre in Surrey, hoping he could be helped to walk again. He was there for a year, and credited a PMRAFNS Sister with getting him mobile again. He told her he lived in a mountain village with steep steps up to his home, so he must be able to walk again.

They always kept in touch, and by the time she was Matron in Akrotiri he was living alone in his own flat. He invited her to his sister's wedding, and as she did not want to drive in the mountains after dark she asked me to take her. The village was remote, on a steep hillside indeed, and the 'steps' up to Varney's house were so high we felt climbing skills were needed rather than walking.

First we attended the ceremony in the village Greek Orthodox church, which included holding crowns above the heads of the bride and groom. Outside afterwards many photographs were taken in the square, then we were taken to Varney's home for a meal.

The only possible access was via the rocky giants, but once there we were given a warm welcome and delicious food. After that we headed back down to the village cinema, an empty, cavernous concrete space. which rapidly filled with wedding guests, music and dancing. Though very crooked, Varney danced! What a joy to see.

An American guest was thrilled; I've no idea who he was but he told me he studied Cypriot traditions (maybe all Greek traditions), but this one was by far the most authentic he had ever attended. Infuriatingly we had to leave before the bride had money pinned on to her wedding dress – and before we could work out whether the bed in the ticket office was to be part of the fun. Matron had arranged to meet the admin officer for a 1.30 am visit (raid!) on the service- women's quarters. Unbelievable. She did regret having fixed it for that night, not realising the celebrations would go on so long, but in all my service I never heard of any other senior officer doing such a nocturnal inspection. I drove back down the mountain roads in a towering rage, going much too fast as we left too late. But I got her there.

Pauline O'Donnell was a QA I knew slightly. She had been the senior midwife in Wroughton, and was fairly notorious as a prickly character. Apparently she had long had an ambition to work at St John's Ophthalmic Hospital in Jerusalem. One day she received two letters, the first promoting her to Lieutenant Colonel, the other offering the post of Matron at St John's. She chose St John's, and was there when I arrived in Akrotiri. After a third message pressing me to visit her in Jerusalem I capitulated, not really difficult as the chance to explore Jerusalem was too good to miss.

One evening in the Mess – the large and only one – no separation of RAF, Army, or female officers, I found myself next to one of the less affable men, but not for the first time with such men found a serious conversation, or at least an ordinary one, was possible. Though I was looking forward to exploring the Old City of Jerusalem, I was slightly doubtful about doing it on my own while Pauline was on duty.

He assured me it would be safe, and added that he had once spent six hours there. I spent seven. Pauline and I got on very well together, and I had a wonderful time.

One day I caught an early morning bus for the three hour journey to the city of Tiberias. What a shock to see young soldiers carrying their weapons casually in the bus station, on their way to catch ordinary service buses to their duty posts. Clueless about politics, it was not until long afterwards that I woke up to the fact that the high chain-link fence on the right-hand side of the road was actually the border of the Left bank. That was the day I bought a paperback book of prayers, treasured ever since, in the Church of Scotland Centre bookshop, and later sat on a low harbour wall watching fish in the Sea of Galilee. Furthermore, I returned to Jerusalem again the following year, and when Pauline came to Cyprus a couple of times for short breaks we met every evening for a meal.

She only liked red wine so we only had red wine. Thanks to her dominance, having until then only liked white wine, I have enjoyed red wine too ever since – and in any case the local Cypriot red was better than the white.

Every autumn, at the end of the grape harvest, there was a major wine festival in a big park in Limassol. On arrival one was given an empty one litre carafe, to be filled as one fancied from any of the main stalls. That night I chose white, took one mouthful and ditched the rest. It was the most lethal alcohol imaginable.

My 50th birthday was in July, six months into my posting, so by then I knew a lot of people and decided to have a party. Easy to arrange as the Mess staff would help with the catering, and everyone could be in the garden or on the veranda.

My decades-old jinx on holding parties vanished in a most unusual mix of guests. Parties were almost a way of life in Akrotiri, but families with small children at the same party as fast jet pilots was unheard of as far as I know. There were doctors, dentists, engineers, admin staff, nurses, helicopter pilots, transport pilots, 100 Squadron 'tow the banner' pilots, and the fast jet ones from whichever squadron was out at the time for its four week training in Cyprus – not least aiming firepower at the banner.

Fast jet pilots are notoriously arrogant. They have good cause to be, so it was a sight to behold watching them play with the children. They chased 3- and 4-year-olds up to my sitting room window, lifting them to feed through to someone inside, then chasing them down the passage to Yvonne's sitting room and out ready to do it all again. It was almost more fun watching the Top Guns than the children. They could let their hair down after all.

My other Top Gun tale illustrates their reputational character. Matron and another PM were going to the station cinema and invited me to join them. When we got there it transpired they had also invited the incumbent fast jet pilots, which is how I found myself sitting next to one. During an interval I offered him some Smarties, which he accepted, so I told him I should evermore enjoy boasting that once upon a time I had fed a Top Gun with Smarties. If looks could kill ... Such an insult to his image! We never encountered each other again, I never knew his name and forget which squadron, so he had no need to be concerned.

Another anecdote about a pilot was nothing to do with me but had become Mess folklore. For our self-service breakfasts a toaster on a side table had become famous. Basically it was a conveyor belt, quite a long one, where a slice of bread fed in at one end emerged precisely done at the other. Very old and prone to breaking down, the engineers were always implored to fix it, because it was unique – and made perfect toast. The RAF pilot of this tale was posted to America, and recorded that he arrived at a big USAF base feeling lonely and a bit apprehensive. Within five minutes of meeting his first US pilot they were sharing happy memories of the Akrotiri toaster. Result! As the young would say.

One of the first things I was told, on being briefed on the ways of Akrotiri, was that flights were sometimes possible. Knowing nothing about planes I asked which was the fastest, but that possibility was doused at once. Lightnings were the fastest but were single seaters. Also, if a rare training two-seater became available, efforts were always made to give the ground crew flights. After that I didn't give flying another thought, but flying more than kindly thought of me.

Apart from the helicopter flight to Dhekelia my first flight was with the Red Arrows! Six of us received invitations, it having been thought a good idea to give a few of the nurses a chance to experience their skills. In every spring the squadron came to Cyprus for pre-season fine-tuned training before authorisation for the display season.

Formalities completed, including approval signatures. a medical, and pre-flight briefings, we rendezvoused at the base beside the runway. First we were kitted out with expert care, given flying suits which fitted well and a helmet so precise that once on my head it was finally adjusted to size using a screwdriver. What a way for my small head to acquire a hat that fitted properly. Next came white gloves, unforgettable because the leather was thinner and finer than any ever seen. (At a party many years later, enthusing about them to a neighbour, he was delighted. He had been responsible to the Air Ministry for finding and acquiring that leather.)

Boots: Tick. G Straps: Tick. Ready: Tick.

Walking out to the runway we passed some trolleys; tall, heavy, double-sided.

Like so much else of this day, an impressive memory, as they were full of tools; shining, immaculate pieces, all looking brand new, hanging in neat rows, engineering an abstract pattern which looked suitable for Tate Modern.

The exercise that afternoon was for each pilot to liaise with the control tower for take off and landing. When formation flying only Red One, the leader, liaised with the control tower, the others just followed him. To maintain their ability each pilot must liaise with the control tower on their own account once a month. This had been explained to us as reassurance, because if anyone felt uncomfortable at any time during the allotted thirty-five minutes they could ask to return to base without upsetting the exercise. However, as all flying time is logged in minutes it would curtail a time entry in that pilot's logbook.

At 'my' Red Arrow – the paint almost rivalling the tools on a scale of shinyness – I was introduced to Dan F., the pilot, then climbed into the back seat of the Hawk. All RAF pilots learn to fly in Hawk jets, they are two seater aircraft, with one behind and quite high, above the other, allowing unimpeded visibility, also the plane has dual controls.

A member of the ground crew strapped me in, fixed a communications headset over my helmet, showed me the eject button while daring me to touch it unless instructed, and I was ready. Dan was soon settled in the front seat, and rather to my surprise I could hear him quite clearly through my headphones. We soon took off, and while airborne I had at least three more surprises. The first was when Dan asked if there was one of the formation manoeuvres I would like to do. Whenever given a chance to choose one of several things my mind goes blank. Some formations are lovely and have attractive names but the only one I could think of was the Bomb Blast. So we did it. Climbed to a suitable height then nose dived vertically.

The second surprise was looping the loop. It was so slow. It was almost as if there was nothing to describe rather than being lost for words. We kept turning without any particular sensation, until the sea appeared above my head looking like blue crinkly tissue paper. It was beautiful, a stunning memory ever since.

The third surprise was the biggest of all. 'Take control, Mary.' I could not believe my ears, but of course did as I was told, even managing two or three small moves, upward, downward and round. Dan said I did well, using a gentle touch which was all that was needed. Largely due to sheer fright actually, but in any case the Hawk was so responsive that gentleness was enough.

Just before this magical flight completed its time allowance I began to feel ready to land, which was irritating, but slight queasiness, and greying out, were uncomfortable. The thought of having to ask to land early was awful, but luckily we were soon down on the runway, and in the general excitement of everyone getting together a couple of quiet minutes was enough to regain my equilibrium. Deeply grateful not to have to tell of feeling peculiar, greying out was nevertheless a bit of a puzzle because I had never heard of it. Probably connected to strong G Forces, but I didn't ask. Long after leaving Cyprus I was reading something a written by a very experienced pilot , and found he had once greyed out, describing exactly what had happened to me. When we were briefed it was never mentioned. Because it is rare or to avoid being alarmist? Never mind. I'd do it all again in a heartbeat.

Following our flights the six of us were taken to the squadron's block, for drinks and reminiscences on their patio, after which I went back to my block and was a zombie for the rest of the evening, reliving all the excitement before going to bed and sleeping for eleven hours.

At the end of their four weeks in Akrotiri the Red Arrows did a special display for the hospital, then shortly after that a final one for assessment; the culmination of all the planning, including new manoeuvres for the forthcoming season. Senior officers flew out from the UK to decide whether the team was good enough to do public displays in the coming summer. Despite what the rest of us saw as perfection, the pilots were keyed up and not taking approval for granted. Hard to believe, but true, and many of us watched with bated breath on their behalf. Fortunately all was well.

100 Squadron was in Akrotiri permanently, its chief roll to tow the banner. In other words, to provide a moving target for fighter pilots to fire at. The banner was analysed afterwards for each pilots success rate; no idea how these were identified individually.

Fighter Squadron detachments came to Cyprus for four or five weeks, usually once a year, because good weather was almost guaranteed. For us it meant a rolling turnover of visiting pilots, with every group keen to host social events and make the most of everything Cyprus had to offer.

One day I was asked if I would like a flight with 100 Squadron. Yes, please! After a briefing, one day I went up in a Canberra, something of a workhorse for the RAF. With a flying suit, 'bone dome' and G Force strap fitted, my seat was next to the Navigator. As warned, there was no view outside, but he explained the many instruments at his desk – a cubby hole in a corner of the fuselage, behind, and out of sight of, the cockpit.

His briefing was so clear it was easy to understand far more than expected of the daunting array of dials and gauges. We heard a couple of shots at the banner, then had to land early as the skipper was not feeling well. So my photo was taken with just the other two crew members, and an apology that there had not been time to give me a turn at the controls.

Part of my initial unhappiness about my posting to Cyprus was a concern about the summer heat. A friend suggested asking for leave in August, which hopefully would give me a fortnight's respite, back home in the UK. Leave in August became leave at Christmas. There were all sorts of delays, not least the terrorist attack and matron away having a knee operation; but from the earliest possible date I had applied for an indulgence flight. By the time I postponed the date for a third time I had a real ally in the station admin office. No idea who she was, but despite the extreme rarity she was determined to try and get one for me.

I was warned near the date deadline that a flight was a near impossibility, so it was a shock to get a phone call telling me there was a stand-by seat available next day. It meant starting my leave a day early, but the CO was delighted for me and readily gave permission.

Which is how I got a flight in a Hercules. They have a notoriously uncomfortable reputation, with the seating being canvas 'bucket' seats slung in metal frames along the side of the fuselage, one row on each side of the plane. On my flight the wide centre space was filled with cargo, including a huge metal container too high to see over the top.

Perhaps because I did not have a parachute strapped to my back the seat, though a bit narrow, was more than adequate. Agreeably surprised by the warmth, earplugs, and food boxes, the only disappointment was having my back to the windows.

But not for long. I was invited up to the flight deck to watch flying over the Alps, and then invited to stay. There was plenty of room to stand in a corner by a window, well out of the crew's way, and there I stayed until we landed. Flying up the English Channel I could see the coasts of England and France both at once – thrilling! A big surprise was seeing what must have been the Goodwin Sands, some distance out from the coast, a long stretch of golden sand, totally out of the water, so it must have been low tide. Next came a perfect view of the White Cliffs of Dover; then the Thames Estuary and the Wash.

We were to land at Coningsby, but suddenly I was asked if I would prefer Lyneham? No contest. 100 per cent easier to get to my sister from Wiltshire than Lincolnshire.

At Coningsby we had to go through Customs, but then some of us boarded again. My main delight was recognising Blenheim Palace as we flew south-west over the Midlands. From Lyneham there was transport to Swindon railway station, which was perfect except that it ran to a timetable and that meant a long wait. At the station RTO office I was given a ticket to Goring, and between changing trains in Didcot there was time to phone and ask, if not too busy, could my brother-in-law collect me at Goring station in half an hour? That was fun as they had no idea I was not in Cyprus.

At the end of leave the civilian flight back was a definite anticlimax. Life resumed its relentless pace the minute I was met after landing in Larnaca. My posting home arrived only three weeks later, though not to be until July, so five months warning. It soon gave me two extra causes for celebration as permission was given for me to drive home from Greece, and to my joy my 12-year-old nephew was to be allowed to fly out to Athens to join me.

With all that to look forward to, three exceptional flights in my last fortnight ended my days with the RAF on a very high note indeed.

The first was in a Shackleton, of 8 Sqn., a plane similar to the wartime Lancasters, those 'four-engine bombers' which enthralled all of us schoolchildren during the war. It was a large, solid aeroplane described by a Warrant Officer as a time warp. The inside was spacious and comfortable, the leather seat coverings were years old. It had a crew of nineteen and even boasted a wardroom. Which is where I sat when first taken on board, and from it had a super view of Akrotiri. My diary is very detailed so will quote it in full.

> Later taken to a high seat near the pilot. Saw Lebanese mountain tops before turning west again. Once I saw two miniscule black dots racing below us; 5 Sqn Lightnings. They were an interesting indication of the distance between us and Akrotiri. I spent ages guesstimating; very difficult, but cheered to be proved right when Dave, the Captain, said we were thirty-seven miles out.
>
> He explained the instruments and showed me an interesting printed plan of the airfield, with radio and landing details.
>
> Suddenly a flurry of voices; 'returning now, no time to give me a go as pilot'. By then I was flat on my tummy in the nose, looking down through the nosecone window, but sadly, as guessed, was not allowed to stay there for landing, had to be strapped into a seat.
>
> I did not eat the snacks or ham salad offered, but was given orange squash and very good coffee. It was a thrill to fly with a window open, lovely air especially as it was a very hot day. Dave was quite right, 'best air conditioning'.

There were two happy postscripts to this flight. A couple of days later an enormous Mess party was held at the Beach club. It was a great evening, with innumerable friends, an early paddle, plenty of good food, with generous bagsful left over, for 'our' two cats, dancing; I danced four times, a few folk swimming, a lot of fun to watch. At midnight I said I would swim if a group would, and one was organised by John D. of 8 Sqn. The challenge was only so that I could boast of a midnight swim, but in fact it was wonderful. Water warmer than expected, and I swam out to a raft. There sat a lone guy enjoying the stars, which were clear and brilliant away from the beach lights. We quietly shared the peace for some time before swimming back together. A few days afterwards he confided that he had told his wife and children about our starlight peace and swim, saying it was something he would remember for the rest of his life. How lovely.

So will I; there was a special feel about it. No hidden agenda, just enjoying the moment. He was Ian Morton of 8 Sqn, and in the middle of an even more frantic day than usual, at Happy Hour 8 Sqn gave me a framed print of a Shackleton, signed by every member of the crew, all nineteen of them. Signed prints like that are as rare as hens teeth, and to be treasured. Mine certainly is. Ian had organised it, and wrote Water Baby under his name. The day of the presentation was the most remarkable of all my days in Akrotiri – more to come about that.

Meanwhile the day before all that excitement, not quite as hectic but memorable nonetheless, there was another incredible event. 10 Port Squadron was actually an Army unit, with a small harbour not far from Cape Gata. I was invited to spend a day on board an Army RCL – Ramped Craft Logistic – awful title. To me, a Second World War girl, a Tank Landing Craft.

For an Army exercise it was to transport a unit of soldiers to Malinda beach, some distance along the coast towards Paphos. A day at sea would be a great treat so I was thrilled.

When Cliff, who overheard the invitation, said 'You don't want to be at sea all day, do you?' I silently disagreed. Cliff was a helicopter pilot in 84 Sqn, also based in Akrotiri. A few months earlier he had married a PM and was a good friend of the hospital. He went on to offer to collect me from the RCL – by winching me up into a helicopter. That was not to be refused despite leaving the RCL early.

On board RCL 105, 'Arromanches' I was spoilt. Taken on a tour of the bridge, crew quarters, engine room; sat in the Skipper's chair – and understood the Radar.

Given a turn at the wheel, given coffee, then found the roof deck. Sun, some mist, and wind which increased to a Force 8 gale. Sea a shining ultramarine. I revelled in it, but we landed some very seasick soldiers at Malinda.

A delicious lunch was cooked on board, followed by the arrival of the helicopter, which apparently had taken half an hour to find us due to the weather. On the rear deck, after some navigating movements to give shelter from the wind, a huge, handsome man landed, gave me a gloriously reassuring smile and handed me a flying suit. If I had been dying of fright that smile from Airload Master Flavell would have saved me. In no time he had me attached and we began to be winched upwards, with me hanging below him but gripped between his knees. When we reached the door his knees bent me into a sitting position; someone behind took my shoulders and slid me inwards on the floor as gently as a basket of eggs. It was a magic experience, recounted many times since, because for anyone in genuine trouble nothing could have been more heartening than my rescuer's smile, and nothing calmer than my recovery despite the gale.

After being landed at 10 Port Sqn. I walked along to Cape Gata to wave to 'Arromanches' as she returned, I went back and greeted her at the jetty, then drove back to the Mess on Cloud nine.

5 Sqn. was rather special, not least as a friend of the hospital. The CO was Andy Williams, whose father was a doctor and had been CO of TPMH in the past. Andy himself became a patient, having bust his Achilles heel during a hockey match; 5 Sqn. v TPMH.

The Squadron flew fast jets, but the pilots were a friendly bunch. We got to know them better than many because they had three detachments to Akrotiri in eighteen months. The last one was rather a time-killing exercise as their Lightnings were about to be retired. Another detachment, 11 Sqn, one evening hosted a cocktail party and BBQ. Behind me in the queue for BBQ food was Andy Williams, who suddenly said, 'You haven't had a flight in a Lightning, have you, Mary?' It was probably the most astonishing thing that has ever been said to me, but I managed to find my voice and say, 'No. Are you offering one?' 'See John' he replied. Flights were so coveted a junior officer was in charge of compiling a list of hopefuls.

At the time Lightnings were the fastest aircraft the RAF had ever had, and more than capable of going through the sound barrier. Normally single seater, each squadron had one two seater aircraft for training, the cockpit just eleven inches wider to accommodate the second seat. So in my first week in Akrotiri I learnt that a flight in a Lightning was out of the question, then in my last week I had one.

It had begun to look as if it wouldn't happen, because a vital piece of equipment was defective. Luckily Ken, the senior engineer officer, was able to get a replacement sent out from the UK as an emergency. A whispered rumour; 'Emergency' not strictly true, but Ken, a very decent man, was determined to get me airborne.

Take-off was earlier than expected, but a phone call from Ops alerted me and after a hasty scramble I arrived at 09.00 as instructed. Minus camera. Bit of bad planning, said Ken, who later appeared with one. When I turned up to have my kit fitted the Corporal looked horrified, but he soon cheered up and did an excellent job, including G-force trousers which had to fit just so. Best now to quote my diary exactly – it was an action packed flight.

Graeme (Smudge) Smith was the pilot, a Scots boy who looks much too young to be a fast jet pilot. Mini bus to the aeroplane; very high cockpit; (one man injured his back badly when the access ladder fell off); narrow seats and no elbow room.

Took off, – could hear my friend Hilary's voice in the Control tower.

We approached Paphos, then up and away.

Given charge of the stick (steering column), Actually was told to take it, then in formal tones "You have control, Mary" **Unbelievable!** It was very smooth and the plane responded to the tiniest move. Stick back to Graeme, we climbed; then down and reached Mach 1.2; 850mph; then went upside down, about G Force 4/5, which did pull and was fascinating.

Given the stick again, then handed it back when time to land. I had asked if there was any chance of going through the sound barrier but was told it was dubious, various factors including air pressure and temperature needed to be right, and probably not favourable this morning.

But we did it! Though, as warned, an anti-climax.

No bang, no particular sound at all, just a slight juddering for a second or two.

Then two Lightnings appeared, one on either side; I could wave to both pilots and Graeme reported 'Passenger enjoying herself'

As well as the query about the sound barrier not being in that part of my diary, neither was a note about Graeme's attitude. On the way out to the plane, and before take-off, he was rather aloof. We didn't know each other, and I had no idea whether he knew that his boss had offered my flight. No matter; returning to the crew room he was a different man.

He confided that many people, including some very senior officers, wanted a flight in a Lightning merely to be able to say they had done one in the fastest jet, little real interest or enthusiasm. He was delighted I had enjoyed myself so much, which of course had been very obvious, and it evidently cheered him that he had been able to give me a good time. How rewarding for him, and for me, more than a good time, an amazing one. Have not enough words to do justice to this great privilege.

I have already told how this incredible day included the Shackleton picture presentation at Happy Hour and the Shakespeare evening at Curium. Luckily it all happened on a Friday, my last in Akrotiri, giving me a chance to wind down, and finish packing over the weekend.

On Monday, after final farewells, I sailed away from Limassol on the ferry bound for Piraeus. It was a perfect July morning, and from the top deck I watched the Shackleton flying in to land, then saw a couple of Lightnings. The ferry sailed quite close to the southern cliffs of the island, and then somewhere near TPMH there was a sudden almighty noise. A jet appeared from above the cliff, but so low it almost seemed to threaten the ship's signal mast. A lot of passengers were on the deck, all looking startled, but I longed to shout 'That was 5 Sqn saying goodbye to me!'

Twelve months later, in Aldershot, one of 5 Squadron's pilots married one of our QAs. At the Reception Andy Williams was at the same table,

and I told him I was big-headed enough to think it had been 5 Sqn.
saying goodbye to me. He just looked at me and said 'Of course.'

HIGH FLIGHT

Oh, I have slipped the surly bonds of earth
And danced the skies on laughter-silvered wings;
Sunward I've climbed and joined the tumbling mirth
Of sun-split clouds – and done a hundred things
You have not dreamed of; wheeled and soared and swung
High in the sun-lit silence. Hovering there
I've chased the shouting wind along, and flung
My eager craft through footless halls of air;
Up, up the long, delirious, burning blue
I've topped the wind-swept heights with easy grace,
Where never lark nor even eagle flew;
And while, with silent lifting mind I've trod
The high untrespassed sanctity of space,
Put out my hand, and touched the face of God.
John Gillespie Magee

Chapter 18

Final Postings and Retirement

Cambridge Military Hospital Aldershot
1987–1991

FROM CYPRUS I was given permission to drive home through Europe during disembarkation leave.

My brother-in-law, who read Greats (Classics) at Oxford, was delighted to allow my 12-year-old nephew, Julian, to join me so that he could see something of Greece. He flew to Athens in the care of British Airways, and on arrival I was called by loudspeaker to reception, where I had to sign for him! From the airport we drove out to Sounion, famous for sunsets, which was indeed beautiful; astonishingly. on the way there we had a ringside view, across a narrow bay, of a seaplane water bombing a forest fire.

After that exciting start in Athens we went to the Acropolis, visited the Parthenon and the nearby amphitheatre. Later we went to Delphi, then down into the Peloponnese to Sparta and Olympia, before catching a ferry from Patras to Italy, where I enjoyed Venice during a second visit,

Julian was disappointed at not having a ride in a gondola – too expensive. The whole journey was great, and it was rewarding to watch Julian change from the apprehensive boy who arrived with concerns about food, fires and goodness knows what, to a confident young man who coped well and enjoyed himself.

After that adventure it was back to work, as Allocations Officer at the Cambridge Military Hospital, Aldershot. I had my own office but liaised with the tutors in the School of Nursing next door, as my job was to ensure that all the student nurses were allocated to wards and departments relevant to their training. For some time I was also acting 2nd Deputy Matron.

It was during this time that my father moved into a care home, my sister and I sold the family home in Oxford and I found, to my astonishment, a lovely flat which I could afford, in Pangbourne. A pleasant town on the River Thames. Some years before, driving along by the river there, I had looked up to a block of flats newly built on the cliff above the road. *How dare they build those modern monstrosities up there* said I to myself. To live in they were very well designed and I was extremely happy. I was allowed to commute to the Cambridge, though always staying in the QA Mess when on call.

From being Allocations Officer I was transferred to the Gynaecological and Ante-Natal clinic, taking over after a much-liked civilian Sister retired. The department was small and cramped, airless, overheated. There were several staff personality clashes and one person in particular caused major problems. She was extremely able, resented a lack of promotion (due to personal problems) and had a huge chip on her shoulder. I failed to cope with her.

My final effort ended with this manipulative young woman complaining to the Midwifery Matron. I was interviewed by an incensed Matron, who calmed down when I explained my side of the story, but I was also interviewed (sympathetically) by the Commanding Officer. The result was my transfer to SCBU (Special Care Baby Unit), with no responsibilities except caring for ill and premature babies.

Ignominious for a senior Major, but it did not rankle. I had never been career minded and retirement was approaching fast. Majors retired at age 55.

However fate had yet another plan. In 1990–91 the UK joined the USA in going to war in Iraq, starting with a brief invasion of Kuwait.

The Cambridge closed all but two wards, and Louise Margaret Maternity Hospital closed completely – sadly never to reopen. Most Departments transferred to the civilian Frimley Park Hospital, a few miles away. Many of our staff were sent off to a two week training camp prior to going to Kuwait and suddenly I was Acting Second Deputy Matron again.

One surprising outcome was having to comfort doctors! In addition to their own personal preparations they had innumerable difficulties with transferring their departments to Frimley Park. There were not even enough desks for the extra offices needed for example, let alone concern about patients and their records.

The invasion of Kuwait was quickly and successfully completed and the left-behind staff were soon welcoming home our returning heroes. After flying back to RAF Brize Norton their buses reached CMH in the middle of the night, so the balloons, music and happy greetings by families and staff were soon over.

The Second deputy Matron also returned, and threw me out of her office, and for my last six weeks in the Corps I did not have a proper job. Matron and others were frantically trying to restart parts of the hospital; it must have been a nightmare. My fate was the least of their worries.

Definitely a career which ended not with a bang but a whimper. My haven was an empty office near the School of Nursing, and I had time to complete a voluntary task. In the Admin corridor of the Cambridge were photographs of every Commanding Officer during the one hundred years of the hospital's existence. Not a name, let alone a photograph, of any Matron was recorded anywhere.

I had undertaken trying to remedy this, and succeeded in finding the names and dates of all the Matrons. An enjoyable and satisfying exercise.

I retired from the Corps on my 55th birthday, 7 July 1991.

Retirement

After leaving the QAs I was unsure about what to do next, not wanting to continue nursing. A post-retirement job interview at the Officers' Pension Society – now the Forces Pension Society, a most friendly and helpful organisation – resulted in a post with the charity Friends of the Elderly.

Ultimately I would be a care home manager in one of the dozen residential homes run by the charity

First I was sent to The Lawn, the home at Honeybourne near Alton, to learn the ropes from the manager, Zuhal Septekin, a Turkish woman and the widow of a British Colonel. She was a very nice person and ideal teacher, so it was a happy time. One day she asked me to collect some holiday photos for her. Boots was doing a promotion which gave railway vouchers for films developed, and I had collected several. Zuhal did not want them but I was able to use them. The eventual outcome was astonishing, but more about that later.

After a spell doing holiday cover for the manager at Woodcote Grove, Coulsdon, I was sent to Wimbledon to be acting manager at the much bigger home there. At the end of nineteen pleasant months I had a phone call telling me that I was to go to Nynehead Court, near Wellington in Somerset. My friend the deputy matron was in the office, and I turned to her with the news, explaining that I was to go as acting manager at first, but to be confirmed as manager after the first few weeks. She was pleased for me and I was delighted at the thought of working in my favourite county, home of my grandparents, and mine, during the Second World War.

My time there began on 28 June 1993. It was a beautiful old house in extensive grounds, a glorious place. A week later a letter arrived which shocked me to the core; in fact it made me feel ill for the rest of the day. Mrs Rumney, the Staff Secretary, wrote that no permanent post was available after the acting manager post at Nynehead Court. Five minutes after reading it the manager who was about to leave told me 'the Hurleys are starting on Monday as trainee managers'!!

A newly retired colonel and his wife, neither of them with any previous care experience, and it later transpired that Mrs Hurley did not want to be a manager. Her husband was to be an Administrative and publicity officer, and he was convinced his wife could, and should, be the manager. When I spoke to Mrs Rumney she flatly denied any suggestion that I had been given to understand I could expect to be confirmed as manager, though my friend heard my reaction to her phone call.

There are two sides to most stories, and there was considerable background to all this. I received a lot of support and sympathy from a surprising number of people but the upshot was that I was made redundant with three months salary. A footnote to this sorry tale: Mrs Hurley never became manager because her husband died suddenly days after I left Nynehead.

My redundancy could not have been better timed. A brilliant coincidence. It gave me three months paid leave to prepare for my wedding. Yes, that is what I said – my wedding!

The railway vouchers from Zuhal's films were almost enough to fund a return journey from London to Aberdeen, and I had a railway warrant left. I wrote to my cousin Mervyn, an old friend and a genealogist, suggesting we 'hie' to Aberdeen for an almost free-travel long weekend, in December 1991, to hunt our Sandilands forebears.

He readily agreed, and we made some interesting discoveries. On a previous visit I had seen Sandilands Drive in the city, in a not very salubrious area. This time we found several connections, especially with King's College, including one of the Founders, named on a stone set in one of the original buildings. Mervyn had been in touch with the college Archivist for some time, so was pleased to go and meet him. Also we had an interesting visit to Craibstone, once a family home and now an Agricultural college. There we were given a friendly welcome, and a photocopy of a sketch of the original house done in the 1700s.

Accommodation problems were neither interesting nor welcome. Never bothering to book ahead myself, instinctively I felt that Mervyn would, but when I asked him he said no, believing that I had. On a mid-week evening in early December a promising B&B I had noted was full. A hunt ensued, taking in everything from a mile long road lined with B&Bs to the poshest hotel in town. Eventually, I offered to pay for a taxi, and with the help of the driver, a hotel with a vacant (double) room was found and Mervyn went to see it. Large, with double beds, but I flatly refused it, dreading what his mother and my sister would say. By now he was incensed because usually he always booked ahead, as I had assumed he would, so obviously I had misheard or misunderstood him.

By now feeling quite dreadful, and with a toxic cousin, the taxi driver drove us to Stonehaven, seventeen miles away, as he knew a pub with good rooms. Unfortunately it was either full or closed, I can't remember which. Eventually, I capitulated and we settled for sharing a double room in the town's biggest hotel.

Far from thinking I was aiming to get my hooks into Mervyn, when my sister heard my reluctant tale she thought it hilarious and so did Mervyn's mother, not least as he had form about sharing a room with a woman. Something to do with a hitch in bookings on a cruise in Egypt, and he offered to help the situation by sharing a night with an American woman. As a shy and faintly eccentric bachelor these episodes did not fit his image at all, but at least our friendship survived.

178

I wrote notes about all the family tree discoveries, and asked Mary, Mervyn's mother, if she thought Pat Sandilands, the family historian, would be interested in them. She gave me his address, in Scotland, and I sent them off to Colonel (Retd.) Patrick Sandilands. His friendly reply included relating an amusing incident at Craibstone when he went there to explore during the war. I replied, and so began eighteen months of correspondence.

He became anxious to meet me, finding mutually convenient dates was difficult, and our letters were getting a bit stilted. At last I went to Scotland in June 1993, stayed on his farm near Oban, for four nights then drove him down to the Borders to stay with his daughter. Madeline, his wife, had died four years earlier, after they had forty happy years together.

When I got up that last morning at the farm, Lagganmore, in lovely Scammadale, I knew we would be married one day. My Highland Grannie's second sight perhaps? Later, I remembered that Pat had dropped a hint the day before, but I thought my imagination was running away with me.

In October Pat came to Pangbourne to stay, so that he could meet my family, and the day after arriving he asked me to think about marrying him. In November I returned to Lagganmore, Pat gave me a beautiful diamond and sapphire engagement ring, a family one, and we went to the *Oban Times* office to arrange an engagement announcement. They offered to send this to *The Times* and *Telegraph* which was helpful, and then we went to the Iona jewellery shop to get my ring altered to fit.

When I left for home, travelling by train, I sat looking at the ring in disbelief, and admiring it for most of the journey. Incidentally, Pat was 82, I was 57, so it was a bit of a nine days wonder for quite a few people, especially in Argyll, where Pat was well known in farming circles, and Madeline had been a Cordon Bleu cook and very sociable hostess. No one had heard of this woman claiming to be a Sandilands!

Pat was born and brought up in England, but his father always insisted that he must remember he was Scottish. He joined a Scottish Regiment and then settled in Scotland. My father merely said that Sandilands was a Scottish name. Interestingly, I felt at home the first time in Scotland, on holiday in Edinburgh in 1958. When Pat and I first met he produced a copy of the Family tree which was identical to the one my father had – a printed one commissioned by my great-grandfather in late Victorian times.

A different coincidence was reading in the *Telegraph*, in the 1960s, of a child bridesmaid called Mary Sandilands. Some forty years later she became my stepdaughter.

Pat was facing a knee replacement operation, and visiting him in hospital I wanted to be his wife, not fiancée. We married in the beautiful church in Checkendon, Oxfordshire, which Jenny and I had known for years, and I was married from her home in the village there; about six miles from Pangbourne.

So on 29 January 1994, on a mild, pleasant winter day, I swopped from Miss to Mrs Sandilands.

For our honeymoon we had a week in Lyme Regis followed by a week in Madeira, but for our first night, fearing we would be tired (which we were) we stayed in a hotel a few miles from Pangbourne,

Next morning we set off to go for a walk but from the main entrance steps noticed our car across the far side of the car park. It looked odd, swathed in something white. On closer inspection we found it completely wrapped in loo paper...

Later we learnt that my highly respectable ex-senior-police-officer uncle, who had given me away at our wedding, had led a family party to the hotel to perpetrate the crime. Almost the funniest aspect was the wooden expression maintained on the face of the hotel doorman as we discovered the joke.

It would be wonderful to say we lived happily ever after, but tragically Pat was found to have cancer of the Parotid gland, at the time of our first wedding anniversary. Even before we were married he used to complain of a dry mouth, and fetch a drink of water, so maybe that was the start of it. With hindsight I was pretty sure he had suffered a lot of pain in silence, being a stoic army officer who among other horrors had suffered an awful time in Italy in 1943/4, enduring an appalling winter in the mountains; extremely cold and with difficult living and supply conditions.

Now, after many weeks spending every Monday to Friday in hospital in Glasgow, he came home for good, and died peacefully on 29 August 1995.

It was expected by some people that I would return to Pangbourne, but I wanted to stay in an area where Pat was known, and hoped to meet his friends with memories of him. I also longed for a view of the sea.

Amazingly, about a year later, I found a bungalow on the Isle of Seil, about six miles from Scammadale, with the sea at the bottom of the garden and wide views across Easdale bay to several islands. Now there for twenty-eight years, I am involved with various local activities, but before telling about them I remembered a holiday with my older niece, which recalled other foreign adventures. So many in fact that they threaten to become a travelogue.

Because Julian had a holiday with Aunty Mary, of course his two sisters had to have the same chance. In 1992 Alison would not choose anywhere, but my ideas led to Boston, USA, which became a flight to New York and a car hire drive north. We visited the Statue of Liberty, went to the top of one of the towers of the World Trade Centre of tragic later memory, then drove up to Boston and onward to Cape Ann. There, from Gloucester, we went whale watching, when we were lucky enough to see a humpback breech six times, coming ever closer to the boat. Thrilling. Other adventures too, so a happy, successful holiday. At the time flights were often overbooked. We volunteered to stay an extra day, were given rooms in a nearby hotel and enough vouchers to enable me to fly back to America the following year, to see the Grand Canyon!

In 1996 younger niece Charlotte chose Egypt, wanting to see the pyramids, but the country was in political turmoil so we went to Mexico instead. A great success, with no end of sight-seeing from Mexico City, via ruins and pyramids – and a tarantula – to Cancun.

Back on the Isle of Seil life involved membership of the RBLS (Royal British Legion Scotland).

Pat was President of the Easdale branch, and it is recorded in the Minutes that when he announced his engagement he said that I would be joining. He hadn't asked me! Years later the Secretary read out that entry at a meeting and we all had a good laugh. It is a happy branch, and for its small size very successful at fund raising for Service charities.

A friend introduced me to the local branch of 'The Rural'; the Womens' Institute of Scotland.

Like the RBLS a happy branch, but skills in crafts are not my forte. She also introduced me to the Argyll branch of the NTS (National Trust for Scotland), which led to hearing many interesting speakers and going on fascinating visits to properties all over Scotland. Every summer we had three days away, with some excellent stays in different parts of the country. Sadly no more; we could not recruit enough volunteers for the committee.

My husband was an Elder in the Church of Scotland, and when he took me to Kilninver village church for the first time I expected an austere service with no music. How wrong I was.

Winnie, our organist, was – and still is – wonderful, able to play any tune. The Minister was young and able; six years later he asked me to be an Elder, saying the Kirk Session had asked for me! Happily we are on good terms with other churches in Oban, especially St John's Episcopal Cathedral.

In 2000 a Slate Islands Heritage Museum was opened in my local village of Ellenabeich. There was an excellent little museum on Easdale Island, a three minute ferry ride from Ellenabeich, but the Trustees felt that a branch on the 'mainland' would be a good idea. For more than 200 years the attractive Bridge Over the Atlantic – proper name the Clachan bridge – has connected the Isle of Seil with the mainland, so much easier access for museum visitors. I am one of several volunteers who do a morning or afternoon stint there, and hugely enjoy meeting visitors from all over the world who find their way to our small corner of Argyll.

Incidentally, for as long as I can remember I have enjoyed bridges, often admiring their architecture and wide variety of styles and materials. Years ago, one day on the ward in Munster, for some reason I said as much to one of our young nurses. She looked at me with sympathetic horror, clearly thinking that Sister had really lost it this time. A week later, on the top shelf of the Red Cross book trolley, was a book about bridges. What's more, the cover photograph was Wallingford bridge over the Thames, a bridge I knew well. Showing it to the sceptical nurse was most satisfying. Vindicated!

In Ellenabeich we have a modern village hall, a much enjoyed hub of our community, used for an enormous variety of events. Music is important in the west of Scotland, and in the hall we have many kinds, from traditional Gaelic choirs and folk groups to classical concerts.

We are lucky in having very good acoustics. So has St John's cathedral in Oban, where every month classical musicians perform, many of them world renowned.

More recently I have joined the Oban U3A, enjoying the monthly talks from a wide spectrum of speakers, and also the variety of poetry chosen by members of the Poetry group.

At home visitors revel in the views from my windows, and for those here on holiday there are innumerable places to explore, both in this area and on the nearby islands. I cherish a memory of attending a NTS Area Committee meeting on the top of Staffa on a glorious June day, climbing up to the plateau complete with brief case (definitely OTT). We sat on the grass in a big circle, my branch report took two minutes and the whole meeting was over in time for us to go down to Fingal's Cave.

A man whose family home was on Mull, but who worked in Edinburgh, had long had an ambition to play his bagpipes in the cave. Not only did he achieve it, he played a composition of his own – and it was his birthday. A joyful experience for all of us.

There are many great places around Oban which are easy to visit. A classic day is one by ferry, bus and boat from Oban to Mull, Staffa and Iona. Iona, St Columba's isle, is beautiful, and many people sense a special atmosphere of peace. Further afield, days out driving to explore many parts of Scotland – Glencoe always terrific – and journeys to family and friends in England have not precluded foreign explorations.

In fact listing them was a shock. There are so many! Far too many for detailed stories, so at the end there is just one, though choosing that has been quite difficult, given many exciting adventures.

USA	Six times. All except one with family members. In 2005 a special highlight was a visit to Massachusetts General Hospital in Boston. Knowing the book 'Sue Barton Student Nurse' off by heart, seeing the Rotunda, an 1840s operating theatre, (now a museum), site of a major episode in the story, was an unexpected treat.
New Zealand	Twice. Did a bungee jump and sky dive.
Greece	Twice
Turkey	Once, sailing with friends.

Switzerland	Twice, to stay with Alison when her husband, Graham, was working near Lausanne.
Vietnam	Once. Terrific tour, including a boat on Ha Long Bay and one on the Mekong river.
Canada	Once. The Rocky Mountaineer train from Vancouver to Banff. Fantastic scenery
France	Once. La Rochelle, with sister and brother in law, to greet Round the World yacht crews.
Italy	Once. To explore Rome.
Czech Republic	Once. To explore Prague
Germany	Once. A long W/E to revisit Berlin.
Argentina	Twice. First, at two weeks' notice, to Buenos Aires to deliver special socks (suitable for the Antarctic Ocean) to my nephew Julian, who was doing the Round the World yacht race. Second, en route to Antarctica .
Antarctica and the Falkland Islands	Once. Exploring on a small ship. Phenomenal. Magical.
Hong Kong	Once. En route to New Zealand, to visit old haunts.
Thailand	Once. Bangkok. En route home from New Zealand.
Uzbekistan	Once. In May this year, 2024, exploring the Silk Road. One of my greatest ever experiences! A steep learning curve, in a lovely group, with good leaders.

This tale is from my first trip to Buenos Aires. The whole idea started as a joke – that I should deliver some socks to Julian, but suddenly I was in a plane flying to South America.

Arrival, immigration etc. was straightforward, then I found the information desk and asked for a hotel. The staff were friendly but concerned, There were two medical conferences on in the city and every type of accommodation almost fully booked. Eventually a room was found for me in a small, once elegant hotel on a main thoroughfare, the Avenue de Mayo.

It was built in 1895, as Buenos Aires developed into a fashionable, sophisticated city, and it retained aspects of that glamorous era. Now somewhat dilapidated, evinced by a hole in my bedroom wall where the bedside light should have been, I loved it; the whole place was full of character, and I think I remember a beautiful fancy wrought iron lift cage – my room was on the fourth floor.

My window had a wide wrought iron balcony which looked out over the Avenue, and from it I watched several parades, including a big Gay Pride one. That was a shock, though amusing, as at the time I had never heard of such a thing.

Every day was packed with interesting explorations of the city, but after only a couple of days. Julian took me to a travel agency which would arrange a flight to Iguazu and a hotel near the falls. The tickets and vouchers would be ready the next day.

Accordingly, next morning I crossed the road of the one way street and hailed a taxi. They were the commonest form of transport; cheap and ubiquitous. On arrival the taxi stopped in another one way street, this time on the opposite side of where I got in. So I paid the driver, then slid across the back seat to get out on to the pavement. A sharp jab in the back of my leg halted me, and to my astonishment a piece of metal, rather like an awl, was sticking out beneath the seat cushion. As it was a puncture wound it did not bleed much, but certainly needed a dressing. The driver seemed unconcerned by the danger in his cab… So nothing to do except get out.

I saw a pharmacy down a nearby road, and on the main road a bank, so decided to go there first, for the cash requested by the travel agent, then the pharmacy. Opened my bag for bank card – no purse! Obviously left on the seat in the taxi as I looked at my leg.

My ability to walk was not affected so I went along to the travel agency. They were wonderful. Workmen in part of the building were sent for, and arrived with some kind of paint, cotton wool, gauze and Elastoplast. Wound dealt with swiftly and with great kindness, but no sign of antiseptic precautions. Julian was phoned at the marina and he arrived to bail me out, paying for the Iguazu trip and giving me cash for taxi back to the hotel. In my room, after luckily finding some snacks for lunch, I unearthed UK phone numbers for cancelling credit cards and went down to the phone in reception.

The instructions defeated me, and I began to get decidedly stressed, as the receptionist (who spoke minimal English), stayed at the back of the office, apparently oblivious of my call for help.

I stood there pondering on what next when the entrance door opened and a man came in. He was waving a card in his hand. the receptionist came to the counter looking happy. He nodded towards me, and the taxi driver produced my purse!! His next passenger had found it, he remembered where he picked me up, and – thanks to the name on the card – phoned hotels in the area until finding mine. He was sorry all the cash had disappeared. His licence hung over the back of the front seat, and I had noticed his middle name was Christian…

The marina where all the race yachts were berthed was some way out of the city centre. My saintly driver took me there – none too happily I sensed, perhaps because he thought a return fare unlikely. However Julian had given me enough cash to tide me over, so paying him was no problem, and I said goodbye with immense thanks and gratitude.

On a wide stretch of grass just inside the gates of the marina a group of people were working on a huge spread out sail. One of them was Julian. Such luck – it was a huge place. So as the driver had come in waving my credit card, so I walked towards Julian waving it.

The happiest thing about it was the effect on *all* the race crews. They were hating Buenos Aires. The marina was miles from anywhere, some of their accommodation was poor, and a corrupt customs had caused big problems with equipment needed for the Southern Ocean. My tale apparently gave a great boost to their morale, and I did become Aunty Mary to a lot of people! I rejoiced in a wonderful ending.

Now I rejoice in so many aspects of life. With minimal health problems, at 88 years old I am indeed immensely blessed.

Easdale
September 2024